Hands on DYSPRAXIA

DEVELOPMENTAL COORDINATION DISORDER

Supporting Young People with Motor and Sensory Challenges

Second edition

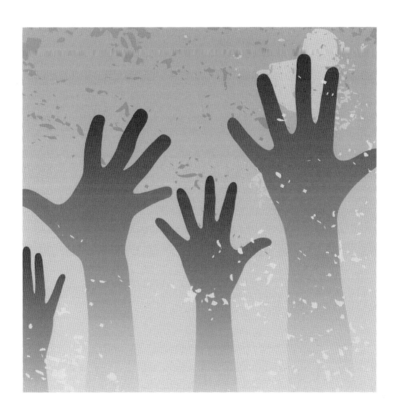

JILL CHRISTMAS AND ROSALINE VAN DE WEYER

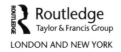

Routledge
Taylor & Francis Group

LONDON AND NEW YORK

Second edition published 2020
by Routledge
2 Park Square, Milton Park, Abingdon, Oxon OX14 4RN

and by Routledge
52 Vanderbilt Avenue, New York, NY 10017

Routledge is an imprint of the Taylor & Francis Group, an informa business

First edition published 2009 by Speechmark Publishing Ltd

British Library Cataloguing-in-Publication Data
A catalogue record for this book is available from the British Library

Library of Congress Cataloging-in-Publication Data
Names: Christmas, Jill, author. | Van de Weyer, Rosaline, author.
Title: Hands on DCD (dyspraxia and allied disorders) : supporting children and young people with sensory and motor learning challenges / Jill Christmas and Rosaline Van de Weyer.
Other titles: Hands on dyspraxia
Description: 2nd edition. | Abingdon, Oxon ; New York, NY : Routledge,
2020. | Revised edition of: Hands on dyspraxia. Brackley : Speechmark,
2009. | Includes bibliographical references and index.
Identifiers: LCCN 2019032776 (print) | LCCN 2019032777 (ebook) | ISBN 9781138600973 (paperback) | ISBN 9780429438998 (ebook)
Subjects: LCSH: Apraxia–Patients–Services for. | Psychomotor disorders in children.
Classification: LCC RJ496.A63 C57 2020 (print) | LCC RJ496.A63 (ebook) | DDC 618.92/8552–dc23
LC record available at https://lccn.loc.gov/2019032776
LC ebook record available at https://lccn.loc.gov/2019032777

ISBN: 978-1-138-60097-3 (pbk)
ISBN: 978-0-429-43899-8 (ebk)

Typeset in Vectora
by Swales & Willis, Exeter, Devon, UK

This handbook is dedicated to my younger sister Sally, who was very involved in supporting children with additional challenges throughout her teaching career. Sally had the idea for the underlying 'hands' design of the original frontispiece in the first edition of *Hands on Dyspraxia*, which is now being carried over to the second edition. She also contributed to the concept of 'What', 'So What', 'Now What' in terms of the book's layout. Latterly, Sally lived with me, following a diagnosis of a severe medical condition, which she fought with her determination and her positive attitude. She is a worthy recipient of this dedication.

Much admiration and our love, Sally (23 June 1952–14 August 2019).

Jill Christmas

Contents

Foreword

Dyspraxia or developmental coordination disorder (DCD) is a common disorder affecting movement and coordination, in which symptoms present in childhood and can persist through to adulthood.

The range and variety of co-occurring difficulties means that the challenges experienced by the individual who presents with DCD often require the intervention of many different professionals in addition to that of the occupational therapist; speech and language therapists, educational psychologists, paediatricians, behavioural optometrists, physiotherapists, teachers and general practitioners, to name but a few. It is therefore critical that all those professionals working in this field, as part of a multidisciplinary team, should have information and training in aspects of this disorder in an effort to offer the best overall intervention possible.

Occupational therapists Jill Christmas and Rosaline Van de Weyer have addressed this need by producing a comprehensive text that can be used by the practising professional. The authors have recognised that the successful management of developmental coordination disorder requires a definition and meaning of the disorder, an explanation of the issues and challenges experienced by the individual, and practical strategies and ideas for intervention, not only for DCD but also for conditions that may coexist with the disorder.

Each chapter follows an easily accessible format, namely 'What', 'So What' and 'Now What', relating to each of the many aspects of the disorder. 'What' comprises an introductory definition and meaning, 'So What' addresses issues and challenges experienced by the individual, and 'Now What' provides practical strategies and ideas for use in treatments. As such, Jill Christmas and Rosaline Van de Weyer have not only offered readers a sound, well- written foundation to the disorder in terms of diagnostic criteria and assessment but have also translated their considerable clinical experience into practical approaches for all professionals working with those individuals who experience developmental coordination disorder. I believe this publication will have a very positive impact on clinical practice and prove a helpful resource for parents and carers.

Stephanie Martin
PhD, MA, Fellow of the Royal College of Speech and
Language Therapy

Preface

The first edition of *Hands on Dyspraxia* was written in 2009, utilising a compilation of knowledge, advice and strategies gained whilst running the Christmas Children's Clinic in Kent and providing comprehensive assessments, reports and therapy.

That book was followed up in 2011 by the publication of *Sensory Dinosaurs*, describing ten fun 'dinosaurs' – each with a different developmental challenge, providing their own story and including an explanation of the condition, strategies and work sheets.

At the end of 2017, I was approached by the publishers requesting a second edition of *Hands on Dyspraxia* relating to current therapy and medical and educational practice. I was on the point of saying no to the project when I was unexpectedly introduced to Rosaline Van de Weyer, principal of Dyspraxia UK in Cambridge. At the first meeting we sensed a shared vision for the new book project and, following further discussion, Rosaline, with her enthusiasm, expertise and willing commitment, confirmed my decision to proceed with the book.

I truly believe that the original book's ethos combined with the current experience and knowledge that Rosaline now brings to this second edition will provide a fresh practical resource supporting professionals working with children and young people.

The original format of the first edition has been re-applied and comprise the following sections:

'What' – What are the challenges the child is presenting with?

'So What' – So what are the implications for the educational, home and social environment?

'Now What' – Now what interventions, strategies and advice are needed to facilitate the child or young person to reach their optimum level of functioning?

Thank you both to Rosaline and the publishers for working so hard to bring this new book to fruition.

Jill Christmas
2019

Chapter 1

Developmental coordination disorder (DCD)

An overview

Developmental coordination disorder (DCD) is also commonly referred to as dyspraxia, by health and education professionals. However, there is a shift to consistently use the term developmental coordination disorder or DCD. This terminology is used for diagnostic purposes and increasingly in both UK and international research literature. The national charity which supports people with dyspraxia/DCD is the Dyspraxia Foundation. They have added developmental coordination disorder to their charity logo to reflect this shift in terminology.

Other terms used to describe developmental coordination disorder may include:

■ Motor learning difficulty
■ Perceptual motor dysfunction
■ Clumsy child syndrome.

These conditions are found in children with intelligence in the average or above average ranges. They can present with relatively subtle symptoms, but often impact on the child's self-esteem and confidence in everyday life. The underlying issues are not easily understood, and they can leave children and adults with a sense of frustration and failure unless they are understood and the right level of support is put in place.

Developmental coordination disorder can be present alone, or be part of a wider neurodiverse profile of overlapping conditions. These are explored in more detail in Chapter 2.

Definition of developmental coordination disorder

The terminology has been a constant source of discussion between professionals, and therefore moves have been made to encourage us to use similar language to improve communication between services.

In 2018, a group of medical and educational experts from the UK agreed a common descriptor of DCD, based on the earlier European Academy of Childhood Disability guidance issued in 2012. The definition is a helpful way of ensuring that all professionals, across health and education, use the same language when talking about DCD in an understandable and accessible way.

This agreed descriptor was presented by Movement Matters, an umbrella group which represents UK organisations with an interest in DCD (see Movement Matters in the 'Professional organisations' section).

UK DCD descriptor (2018) as presented by Movement Matters

Developmental coordination disorder (DCD), also known as dyspraxia in the UK, is a common disorder affecting movement and coordination in children, young people and adults with symptoms present since childhood.

DCD is distinct from other motor disorders such as cerebral palsy and stroke and occurs across the range of intellectual abilities. This lifelong condition is recognised by international organisations including the World Health Organisation.

A person's coordination difficulties affect their functioning of everyday skills and participation in education, work and leisure activities. Difficulties may vary in their presentation and these may also change over time depending on environmental demands, life experience and the support given. There may be difficulties learning new skills.

The movement and coordination difficulties often persist in adulthood, although non-motor difficulties may become more prominent as expectations and demands change over time.

A range of co-occurring difficulties can have a substantial adverse impact on life including mental and physical health, and difficulties with time management, planning, personal organisation and social skills.

With appropriate recognition, reasonable adjustments, support and strategies in place, people with DCD can be very successful in their lives.

To help you understand the assessment process, it is useful to be aware of the diagnostic criteria that professionals use when assessing children and adults, who present with symptoms associated with developmental coordination disorder.

Diagnostic criteria

There are two principle reference points for making clinical diagnoses for DCD. The *Diagnostic and Statistical Manual of Mental Disorders*, 5th Edition, by the American Psychiatric Association (2013) and the World Health Organisation's *International Classification of Diseases* (*ICD*), 11th edition (2018). The content is complementary.

The *DSM-5* diagnostic criteria for developmental coordination disorder (American Psychiatric Association, 2013)

A. Motor performance that is substantially below expected levels, given the person's chronologic age and previous opportunities for skill acquisition. The poor motor performance may manifest as coordination problems, poor balance, clumsiness, dropping or bumping into things; marked delays in achieving developmental motor milestones (e.g., walking, crawling, sitting) or in the acquisition of basic motor skills (e.g., catching, throwing, kicking, running, jumping, hopping, cutting, colouring, printing, writing).

B. The disturbance in Criterion A, without accommodations, significantly and persistently interferes with activities of daily living and/or academic achievement.

C. Onset of symptoms is in the early developmental period.

D. The motor skill deficits are not better explained by intellectual disability (intellectual development disorder) or visual impairment and are not attributable to a neurological condition affecting movement (e.g., cerebral palsy, muscular dystrophy, degenerative disorder). The disturbance is not due to a general medical condition (e.g., cerebral palsy, hemiplegia, or muscular dystrophy).

ICD-11 diagnostic criteria for developmental motor coordination disorder (6A04) (World Health Organisation, 2018)

Developmental motor coordination disorder is characterised by a significant delay in the acquisition of gross and fine motor skills and impairment in the execution of coordinated motor skills that manifest in clumsiness, slowness, or inaccuracy of motor performance. Coordinated motor skills are substantially below that expected given the individual's chronological age and level of intellectual functioning. Onset of coordinated motor skills difficulties occurs during the developmental period and is typically apparent from early childhood. Coordinated motor skills difficulties cause significant and persistent limitations in functioning (e.g., in activities of daily living, school work, and vocational and leisure activities). Difficulties with coordinated motor skills are not solely attributable to a disease of the nervous system, disease of the musculoskeletal system or connective tissue, sensory impairment, and not better explained by a disorder of intellectual development.

Inclusions:

- Orofacial motor coordination disorder

Exclusions:

- Abnormalities of gait and mobility
- Diseases of the musculoskeletal system or connective tissue
- Diseases of the nervous system

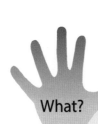

Developmental coordination disorder (sensory motor)

What: definition and meaning

Developmental coordination disorder has been perceived as being due to immaturity of the brain processes resulting in poor organisation, and it can impact on virtually every area of life. It has been suggested that up to one in ten of the population may have dyspraxia or an overlapping DCD.

There are three main components of developmental coordination disorder:

1 **Ideation** – the ability of the brain to think about, or conceptualise what the body needs to do (which should become automatic once a skill is learned). The child with DCD may have to cognitively work out which action is needed each time even though they have performed the action previously.

2 **Motor planning** – the ability to organise one's body for action without having to think about it. With DCD, the child has to consciously think actions through, sometimes at the expense of the task in hand.

3 **Execution** – the ability to respond to input from the environment and make the right movement – in technical terms this is called a 'motor adaptive response' – something that we learn to do from the moment we are born in response to incoming stimuli from around us. Practice refines the movement, and it is then utilised without conscious monitoring.

Young people with DCD tend to exhibit poorly integrated reflexes and postural reactions.

Sometimes immature whole movement patterns adversely affecting gross and fine motor skills can be observed. Children who are often missed, or diagnosed later in life, exhibit a lack of coordination and integration of both sides of the body, this is sometimes referred to as bilateral integration sequencing.

Our sensory systems inform our motor systems; therefore DCD may result from challenges in correctly processing sensory information through our different body 'senses' in order to give an appropriate physical response. The following systems are involved:

■ Balance (vestibular) systems based in the middle ear
■ Body movement and body position awareness feedback (proprioception)
■ Auditory (listening and hearing)
■ Vision (looking and seeing)
■ Tactile (touch sensation)
■ Gustatory and olfactory (taste and smell).

All of the above systems need to function at their best, in order for us to organise our body for use and respond appropriately to our environment. With DCD the senses do not always feed back the correct information, and therefore the child lacks 'sensory integration' and their physical (motor) responses are likely to be compromised.

So
what?

So what: issues and challenges

◆ The child is of average or above average intelligence.
◆ Motor milestones may be within average range, but crawling may be missed out or an unusual crawling pattern such as 'commando' or 'bottom shuffling' can occur; walking may be early.
◆ Muscle tone and strength may be weak, affecting sitting, standing and moving, and the child tires easily as extra effort is required to counter gravity.
◆ Joints may also be lax or 'hyper-mobile', causing decreased stability in trunk, limbs and hand control. The child may experience discomfort in back and neck and when writing for extended periods.
◆ Accident proneness and the tendency to bump into, fall over and knock against objects is common. Objects are knocked over or easily dropped as the child does not always 'register'

the force they are using due to poor sensory (touch or body awareness) feedback (see spatial awareness below).

◆ The child may lack awareness of the position of their arms and legs in space when outside their field of vision (spatial awareness).

◆ New activities may be difficult to learn and more time is needed to acquire new skills (ideation).

◆ Articulation and oral (mouth) motor skills may be poor, and the child's speech may be hard to understand; they may also have difficulty chewing and swallowing food. Meals may be a messy business as the child cannot monitor their movement and hand and mouth coordination outside their visual field when taking food to the mouth.

◆ Dressing may be difficult and clothes tend to be untidy, poorly tucked in and disorganised due to a reduced sense of their body scheme and poor registration of touch. Buttons and fasteners are difficult to do up due to impaired manual dexterity and manipulation, and reduced touch and movement feedback.

◆ Swimming may be difficult (the child's face may end up underwater when flexing arms in breast stroke due to the retained linked movements between head and arms). Skipping and reciprocal cross-pattern movements can be a problem, again due to a lack of integration of both sides of the body.

◆ The child who does not register touch in the usual manner may overreact to simple touch due to hypersensitivity, or alternatively not register pain or discomfort in the usual manner and appear stoic. (Touch registration may also vary in the same child.)

School

◆ In school the child may find it difficult to maintain an upright position at the desk despite reasonable muscle tone. They tend to 'slump' over the desk, lean their head onto their arms, or 'head prop' on one hand at the expense of steadying or stabilising their work.

◆ The child may be uncomfortable sitting in a flexed position at the desk, fidget and experience a loss of concentration. They may tend to sit with legs twisted around chair legs at the desk, prefer to sit on their feet on the chair or alternatively lean back, stretching their arms and legs out in front of them in an effort to feel 'mechanically' comfortable.

◆ When writing or drawing the child may shift their body to the left or right on the chair, turn their body or rotate their paper when drawing across their body midline, due to poor integration between the two sides of the body – the lack of bilateral integration hinders the child from working across the midline of their body.

◆ Associated mouth (overflow) movements may be noted when undertaking resisted manual tasks such as cutting and writing.

◆ The above characteristics can indicate retention of the primitive or 'baby' reflexes which cause immature whole movement patterns. These in turn can limit the child's refinement of their arm and hand control (see the sections on symmetrical and asymmetrical tonic neck reflexes in Chapter 7).

◆ The child may hold the pen in an immature grip with the thumb lapped across the shaft of the pen as opposed to a tripod grip with the fingers on the barrel of the pen; in tandem with retained whole arm movement patterns, this can cause fatigue when writing for extended periods. The child may revert to printing letters as they lack the refined intrinsic finger and thumb movements for cursive formation of letters.

◆ The child may be unsure which is the stabilising hand and which the leading hand, as they may have an unclear hand dominance and change hands depending on the nature of the activity.

◆ Two-handed activities may be difficult to coordinate, including the use of knife and fork, buttons and laces. The child may tend to use whole arm movements with elbows elevated in the air when cutting up food or using scissors.

◆ Some letter reversals may be noted, and dyslexic tendencies are not uncommon in children and young people with an underlying DCD.

◆ The child may have difficulty in keeping their eyes fixed on a moving object in the vertical and horizontal planes, or in looking up to the board and back to their work when copying, and blurring may occur. The child may blink their eyes as an object crosses in front of the midline of their body when asked to visually fix on or track a moving object in the horizontal plane. This may affect smooth eye movement for reading. The child may also complain that their eyes tire although their general vision has been checked and noted as within the norm.

◆ There may be visual perceptual challenges which need to be more formally identified. For example, the child may have difficulty in working both eyes together for binocular vision, and interpreting information such as recognising and matching a shape in a cluster of other shapes. This may be caused by poor 'depth perception' or figure ground recognition.

◆ Balance may be poor with a resulting reluctance to engage in balance related activities in physical education (PE). The child may be fearful of heights, for example.

◆ The child may generally coordinate movements well when activities such as throwing and catching are directed to the middle of the body. They may also excel in a variety of preferred sports, but find cross-pattern movements challenging as this requires integration of the left and right sides of the body.

◆ The child with DCD can find it difficult to organise themselves and their belongings and forget what they were supposed to be doing.

◆ Short-term memory may be poor, instructions difficult to recall, and the child may appear lazy when in reality they are experiencing difficulty translating instructions into action.

◆ Concentration in class may be compromised with loss of focus, particularly when the child's body position awareness (proprioception) is low. They may need to fidget and move around on their seat to maintain physical alertness.

◆ Social skills may be challenged due to a lack of confidence and self-esteem and resulting awkwardness. The child may be reluctant to engage in anything new, causing social isolation.

Now what?

Now what: practical strategies and ideas

Developmental coordination disorder is movement based, and a screening assessment and development programme are normally required under the direction of an occupational therapist to advise upon and support the identified areas of strengths and challenges. Note also the strategies in the handwriting and visual motor integration sections in Chapter 4 and the bilateral integration section in Chapter 6.

Postural support should be provided for extended periods of sitting. Ensure that the desk is at least elbow height, and ideally the surface at a 20-degree angle for school and homework (angled board or file placed appropriately). The chair height should allow feet to be placed firmly on the ground to offer stability and 'sensory' (proprioceptive) feedback.

- Always seat the child facing the focus of the teaching, limiting the necessity to twist and turn; this also allows a 'multi-sensory' approach to teaching – looking, hearing and also observing the teacher's 'body language'.
- Place the child in class where focus can be maintained at the best level – keeping out of the way of main circulation areas assists focus.
- Whole class teaching is ideal, enabling a multi-sensory method of information processing during the lesson and maximum concentration.
- Handwriting difficulties are very common. In class ensure that there is adequate space for forearm support at the desk when writing or typing. Use of textured inbuilt moulded pen grips providing touch feedback and easing of pressure on the pen will assist.
- The child will require strategies in place to assist organisation – see the section on organisation and sequencing skills in Chapter 6. Give the child the opportunity to plan and organise belongings ahead of time, and provide a visual timetable where it can be seen easily and replicated at home and school. Give a two-minute warning for any transition to allow closure of the existing task.
- Ensure that the child with poor ideation and planning has good peer support in the playground and in class. Provide positive feedback for effort made as opposed to the result. Give them personal responsibility for a manageable and regular task which fits in with their personal strength to build their self-esteem.
- Overlearning of motor skills may be required and opportunities for a subtle differentiation in physical education (PE), games and allied activities. 'Splinter' (isolated) skills may be acquired when the child is motivated, but most activities will require extra practice until 'laid down' in the long-term memory part of the brain.

- Exercises should be advised by an occupational therapist to facilitate integration of both sides of the body and upper and lower body movement patterns, and to assist reciprocal and cross-pattern movements. See additional strategies in the bilateral integration section. Exercises then can be integrated into PE classes for the primary school child.

- Ensure that staff are aware that the child may overreact to pushing and nudging if 'touch sensitive'. Place them at the beginning of a queue or where contact is less likely to occur.

- Alternatively, if the child has a reduced sense of touch, check for any injury in contact sports such as football or rugby to ensure safety as they may lack awareness of injury incurred. Also monitor the amount of force a child with DCD uses as they may unwittingly use excessive pressure because of reduced sensory feedback.

- Monitor for joint laxity as a child with weaker muscle tone may be more vulnerable to injury and should not be put in a position of heavy weight bearing – as, for example, in rugby and heavy lifting and handling.

- Advice from a speech and language therapist may be needed to assess and facilitate the child's oral, expressive and eating skills.

- A comprehensive assessment may be sought from an occupational therapist who can advise both the parents and the school on the child's individual sensory and motor needs to provide practical strategies and intervention.

- Allow movement opportunities in the classroom: for example, allow the child to hand out information and provide intermittent short movement breaks to limit 'mechanical discomfort' when sitting for extended periods.

- Additional exercises are recommended to enhance the child's ability to work and write across their body midline. This will enhance the child's ability to sit at the desk without twisting and turning. Whole movement patterns can be reduced by exercises to help the child isolate shoulder, forearm, wrist and finger/thumb movements under the direction of an occupational therapist.

- A programme of reflex integration exercises may provide positive results – see the sections on the symmetrical and asymmetrical tonic neck reflexes in Chapter 7.

- An evaluation by an occupational therapist for handwriting, visual motor and visual perceptual skills can assist in identifying the primary issues and how to address them.

- Refine hand control with specific exercises to promote a tripod grip and provide handwriting programmes if the child is still at primary stage.

- Enhance functional vision with exercises under the direction of an optometrist. Advice should be obtainable in the UK from opticians working under the National Health Service. In addition, advice can be obtained from the British Association of Behavioural Optometrists (BABO – see the 'Professional organisations' section). Other countries will have their own specialists and professionals who can advise on different aspects of the child's eyes.

Oral motor coordination disorder

As highlighted in the World Health Organisation's diagnostic criteria (*ICD-11*), orofacial motor coordination disorder is included under the umbrella of developmental coordination disorder.

What: definition and meaning

■ Oral motor coordination disorder is primarily a 'motor planning' speech disorder and usually has its basis in an underlying developmental immaturity affecting the child's ability to express words in an orderly and sequential manner. The child may have the ideation of what they want to say but not the ability to 'motor' plan and execute the spoken word effectively.

■ Oral motor dyspraxia can also affect the coordination of the child's facial, mouth and tongue muscles, which is required for them to speak and articulate what they want to say in an intelligible and clear manner. Especially if the child is tired.

So what: issues and challenges

◆ The child may find it difficult to coordinate their mouth and tongue movements, and their resulting speech may be unclear and hard to understand.

◆ The child may have had difficulty in copying sounds and early words as a baby and toddler, although they may have the right intonation and speech patterns.

◆ The child may have difficulty in the sequencing and organisation of speech and the ability to get the words out in the correct order despite reasonable listening skills and knowing what they wish to say.

◆ The younger child may use other forms of communication such as sounds and gestures and may not use words or verbalise speech correctly.

- Vowels and consonants may be unclear – especially at the beginning and end of words.
- The child may have indistinct speech and lack confidence in speech production and self-expression. As a result, they may be unwilling to participate vocally in class.
- As the child with dyspraxia is often of average or above average intelligence, the above issues may engender frustration and reinforce a sense of low self-esteem.

Now what: practical strategies and ideas

Now what?

- Unless support and practical intervention are undertaken by a speech and language therapist or speech pathologist, the child may continue to struggle throughout their lives with their expressive speech.
- With applied individualised speech and language therapy programmes, many of these children may learn to speak more clearly and appropriately.
- An occupational therapist with knowledge of this area can also support a speech and language programme with the introduction of a range of therapeutic activities, such as blowing and sucking games, which can be integrated into the child's playtime at school and home.
- It is important to encourage the child to participate verbally in class, providing they are given time to organise their thoughts and allowed to speak without pressure.
- Positive feedback for the effort made is vital, and the child's self-esteem and confidence should be supported at all times – the child may appear 'slow' to those around them and thus their skills and abilities underestimated.
- It is particularly important for a child with oral motor dyspraxia to be helped to identify their interests and strengths so that they are able to shine in at least one area. These children may be late developers, and need the opportunity to find different methods of expressing their intelligence and creativity.
- As these children are normally of average or above average intelligence but struggling with speech and usually written output, a full assessment and evaluation of their overall needs

can be undertaken by an occupational therapist and/or an educational psychologist to identify their strengths and support their challenges.

Sensory motor development in childhood

The 'Christmas' tree (Figure 1.1) illustrates the sensory motor developments that occur in childhood. Developmental coordination disorder can impact upon any aspect, which means that children with DCD will present differently: with differing strengths and challenges. Hence, an individual approach for support is required.

*The
'integrated' child –*
emotional, psychological,
physical, cognitive, spiritual

Gross and fine motor tasks refined

Maturation of personal independence,
behaviours, imagination, cognition, social
and language skills

Functional and physical performance integrating

Eye/hand co-ordination, hearing, attention, information
processing, concentration, visual-motor, receptive, executive
skills maturing

Thinking, organising and 'doing' – ideation, planning, execution

Body control, position awareness and posture control maturing

Sensory systems (hearing, touch, vision, smell, taste) integrating
and fine tuning

Reflex patterns still emerging, maturing and integrating

Body position awareness
Balance
Hearing
Touch
Vision
Smell
Taste

Birth of the baby

Automatic perception of body
scheme (proprioception)

Balance (vestibular system)

Primitive 'baby' reflexes/reactions

Touch (tactile system)

Growth of the baby in the womb

Figure 1.1   The 'Christmas' tree: an overview of early sensory
motor development in the child

The role of the occupational therapist working with children and young people with developmental coordination disorder

Occupational therapists are skilled to actively contribute to the diagnostic process of DCD in young people. A multidisciplinary team assessment is best, given that it is imperative a medical doctor can rule out any other conditions which may account for the symptoms observed. Service provision for this type of multidisciplinary assessment for DCD varies across the UK, so do check with a general practitioner (GP).

Occupational therapists provide a comprehensive assessment of the child and can provide follow-up recommendations in report format with strategies for the child in their daily life, as well as within the school setting. Therapy may also be provided to address the highlighted needs of the child. An occupational therapist may or may not be a specialist in developmental coordination disorder and allied neurodiversities, but if so, is in an excellent position to evaluate the child's strengths and challenges in order to provide understanding and practical support. Close liaison with school staff, feedback from parents and the issues raised by the child him/herself all contribute to gaining a comprehensive profile prior to a full assessment. The following assessment tools are some of many which may be utilised by the occupational therapist to provide a practical and useful profile of the child with DCD:

■ Clinical observations – including the child's engagement with the environment, balance systems, postural strength and stability, ocular (visual) motor skills, body position awareness, coordination of the two sides of the body, tactile skills, eye, hand and ear preference, fine motor control, oral motor skills, presence of aberrant reflexes and sensory issues.
■ Observations and feedback for activities of daily living or life skills – for example, dressing, knife and fork use, bathing, sleeping and toileting issues.

■ Evaluation of physical skills screening using standardised tests, to include large motor movements, manual dexterity, static and moving balance, ball and targeting skills, among others.

Standardised tests

Standardised tests enable the child's skills to be evaluated in comparison with other children of his/her age. The test results enable the occupational therapist to see exactly where the child's strengths and challenges lie, so that specific recommendations can be made to support.

■ Standardised tests of visual motor integration – testing the combined skills of visual perception and motor recording using the medium of paper (handwriting) or technology.

■ Standardised visual perception testing, which includes the more cognitively based skills of visual memory and visual sequential memory.

■ Standardised motor coordination assessment to test: fine motor skills, precision skills, dexterous two handed tasks, static and dynamic balance and strength.

■ Sensory profiling to evaluate the child's level of response to environmental stimuli and the impact they may have on their functioning within the classroom or at home.

■ A range of assessment tools to help the child and the parents evaluate the child's performance strengths and challenges.

A child with developmental coordination disorder may or may not have been assessed by one or more other professionals with whom the occupational therapist may liaise, with the parents' consent, to gain a fuller picture of the child's requirements. For example:

1   Paediatrician and/or general practitioner
2   Teacher/SENCo (special education needs coordinator)/inclusion lead/learning support assistant in the UK
3   Speech and language therapist (SALT)
4   Physiotherapist
5   Educational psychologist

6   Child and adolescent mental health practitioner
7   Optician/behavioural optometrist
8   Audiologist
9   Dietician.

Examples of allied professionals who can support children with developmental coordination disorder

The list below is advisory only. It is the responsibility of the child's parents or carers to ensure that the consultants are formally registered health or allied health professionals with experience in the identified area of concern. See the 'Professional organisations' section at the end of this book.

Speech and language therapy may be recommended for:

- Children with oral motor dyspraxia (difficulty with muscular control in forming words, chewing and eating, for example).
- Assisting and advising on auditory processing and organisation of spoken information.
- Children with heightened 'gag' reflexes and allied sensory issues.
- Verbal/speech output and the ability to organise thought processes into the spoken word.

Physiotherapy may be recommended for:

- Assessing the child's postural control, balance and related issues which may be contributing to their developmental coordination disorder challenges.
- General muscle strengthening and building up of core trunk, shoulder and hip stability.
- Inhibition of poorly integrated reflexes: for example, the asymmetrical tonic neck reflex.
- Gait 'walking' patterns.
- Specific exercises for joint hypermobility.

Educational psychology may be recommended for:

- Gaining an overall profile of a child's cognitive and academic strengths and challenges in relation to their schooling and home for reading, spelling, maths, and handwriting.
- Advice on emotional and behavioural issues, and self-esteem.

- Advice on schooling and placement for a child requiring additional support – including learning support, and liaison between home and school.
- Monitoring and reviewing of the child's progress to help them maximise their academic ability.

Mental health support may be recommended for:

- Self-esteem issues and supporting confidence around self-worth.
- Advice on emotional and behavioural issues, and self-esteem.
- Symptoms including poor sleep, changes in appetite, decreased socialisation, appearing withdrawn, changes in overall mood and self-harm.
- A referral to the Child Adolescent Mental Health Service may be required.

An audiologist may be recommended for:

- Children who have received a hearing test by a medical doctor, but may continue to not hear certain sounds or frequencies, or screen out background noises easily.
- Assessment of auditory processing to see if any frequencies are being missed.

A behavioural optometrist is recommended for:

- Children who are struggling to get their eyes working together to focus and track efficiently. This is essential for copying from the board at school, handwriting and hand–eye coordination for sports.
- Specific exercises to support the muscles surrounding the eyes to enable them to work smoothly together.

A dietician or nutritional therapist may be recommended for:

- Immune system damage which can result in chronic ear infections, asthma, eczema and allied conditions.
- Digestive system imbalances.

■ Eating disorders. Nutrition and supplements are important for brain maturation, in tandem with essential vitamins and minerals to counter toxicity and balance any shortfall, and to optimise the child's overall health and integration.

Chapter 2

Other conditions that can coexist with DCD/ dyspraxia

There are a range of specific learning differences which can coexist with developmental coordination disorder:

- Developmental coordination disorder (DCD) also known as dyspraxia
- Dyslexia
- Dyscalculia
- Attention deficit disorder (ADD)
- Attention deficit hyperactivity disorder (ADHD)
- Autistic spectrum disorders (ASD)
- Developmental language disorders (DLD).

Neuro-diversity is a wonderful umbrella term which describes the range of differences in individual brain function and behavioural traits, regarded as part of normal variation in the human population. Human beings are naturally neuro-diverse, which is indicated through our day- to-day needs and preferences.

Nevertheless, it is helpful to have a diagnostic assessment and subsequent diagnostic label if a child or young person *is observed to be* at a significant disadvantage in comparison with their peers in a learning, home and future work environment. A recognised diagnosis, guides professionals and families to specific resources and support that may be otherwise unavailable.

Specific learning differences of any sort can also impact upon sensory sensitivities (that is, over- or under-responsivity when registering incoming stimuli from either their own body and/or the environment). A young person may also present with social communication challenges.

It is imperative to note that neuro-diversity may also enable a person to be particularly gifted in one area or another. Many of our great thinkers, business people and performers are known to have a specific learning difficulty, as outlined above.

Humans, thankfully, do not fit neatly into diagnostic boxes, therefore in order to obtain personalised recommendations and support, health and educational assessments should be centred around the young person. It is important to be guided by the child and their families as to what their needs are, and to identify which interventions will make the most difference to their lives.

People with any form of neuro-diversity experience strengths and challenges in different areas of functioning, many of which may not be immediately apparent but which may have an adverse impact on their overall functioning. That is why an individualised approach is essential, rather than one that is condition-focused.

Common challenges, may include:

- Over- and under-responsivity to sensory stimuli
- Low self-esteem, mood disorders, depression
- Lack of concentration
- Movement-seeking behaviour
- Distractibility or lack of focus
- Speech/language problems.

Nevertheless, specific learning difficulties of any sort often bring a new, refreshing perspective to tasks and situations. There are many positive role models past and present such as Walt Disney (pioneer of the animation industry), Jamie Oliver (chef and restaurateur), Richard Branson (entrepreneur), Daniel Radcliffe, Orlando Bloom and Keira Knightly (actors), Holly Willoughby and Chris Packham (television presenters), Wolfgang Amadeus Mozart (composer), Albert Einstein (scientist) and Temple Grandin (prominent spokesperson on autism), to name a few.

These prominent role models have different areas of brilliance. Innovation and creativity feature, as does lateral thinking and learning by doing – actively performing and refining tasks and skills.

Dyslexia

This condition can be part of an overlapping profile in tandem with developmental coordination disorder (DCD), or a standalone depending on the underlying cause. There can be a range of contributory factors: for example, dyslexia may arise from visual processing difficulties or from hearing/auditory challenges. Also, dyslexia is not uncommon in children who have immature balance (vestibular) systems, adversely affecting their orientation in space – both for their own body position and for activities such as recording information on paper.

Example: The text in Figure 2.1 was written by a child of 8 years of age. It demonstrates 'mirror' writing, which may be observed in older children who have visual processing challenges and maybe part of the dyslexic profile after the age of 7 or 8.

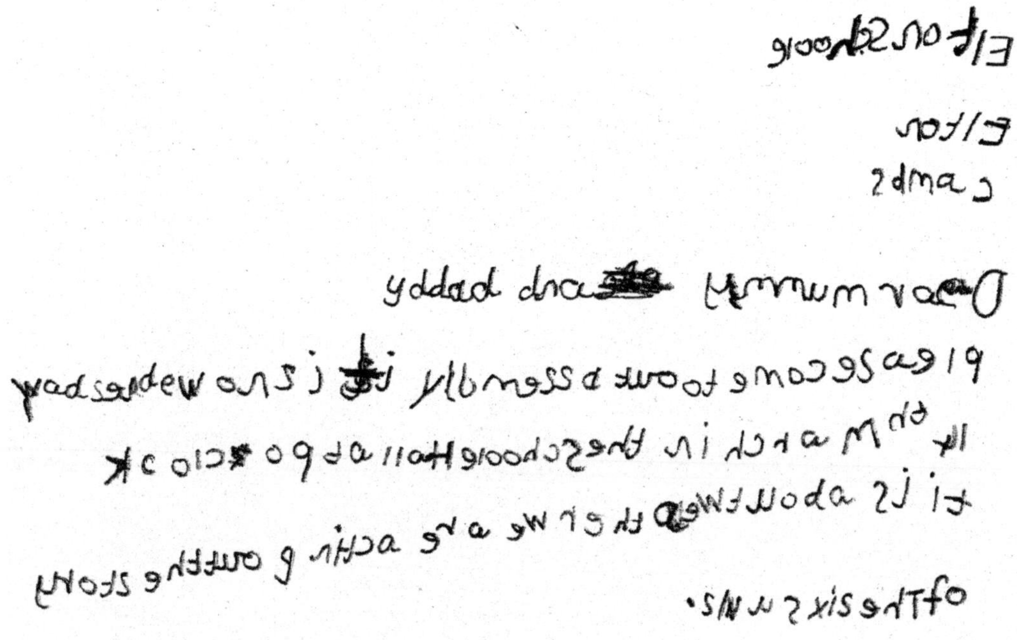

Figure 2.1   An example of 'mirror' writing

This child has written an invitation to her parents, inviting them to attend a class assembly on Wednesday 14th May in the school hall at six o'clock.

Indicators for the child with dyslexia

- Familial history of reading, handwriting and allied challenges are sometimes seen.
- 'Jumbled up' or muddled words and phrases.
- Finds spatial concepts such as left, right, up and down difficult: may reverse letters and numbers or tend to lose direction when drawing or writing on paper.
- May be a very intelligent, a creative thinker and have lots of ideas but has difficulty in getting information down on paper.
- Can be good at concepts with constructional toys but maths may be difficult, for example, with memory sequence or position of numbers and symbols on paper.
- May like being read to but less keen to read or work with letters and words.
- Finds rhythm and rhyming difficult – action songs and nursery rhymes are hard to learn in the early years.
- Difficulty with following a sequence in an activity such as threading beads and recalling what comes next. Short-term recall of information may also be difficult.
- May have motor coordination challenges – for example, a tendency to trip and fall due to a reduced sense of where their body/limbs are in space, or have poor 'saving' reactions (unable to put their arms out in time to save themselves when falling over).
- May lack integration of both sides of the body (bilateral integration) and not have a clearly dominant hand, resulting in difficulty working and writing across their body midline, which in turns causes shifting around on a chair.
- May not have crawled, in part due to retained reflex activity which can 'block' some developmental milestones.

Indicators of dyslexia at primary stage

- Innate and original ideas are hard to get down on paper (although this and other aspects may also be seen in children who are relatively young for their school year).
- May use an immature 'palmar' (whole hand) grasp when using a pen.

- Letter and number reversals are still evident after the age of 7 with directional confusion when changing direction on paper such as when drawing an angled shape.
- Time telling and general time management may be difficult.
- Instructions may be difficult to follow.
- Organisation and sequencing an action or activity can be an issue.
- May constantly forget and need to be reminded of what has been asked of them.
- May lose equipment, forget books and find planning difficult.
- Large and fine motor skills may be difficult.
- As handwriting output increases, there may be an increasing reluctance to write more than a sentence or phrase when asked to write about a topic.
- Frustration, loss of self-esteem and resulting behavioural issues may be apparent.
- Can be verbally able but work output is poor.

Indicators of dyslexia at secondary stage

- Some of the above issues as in primary school.
- School performance and output does not reflect the child's innate ability.
- Reading and sometimes comprehension may be an issue – may be reluctant to read.
- May have functional eye problems – for example, when copying information from a board they cannot maintain line position when writing, and blurring may occur or double vision.
- Difficulty taking down information when dictated by the teacher. Visual sequential and auditory sequential memory is often poor, with the resulting lack of ability to hold a sequence of information in their working memory.
- Difficulty in setting out work logically and methodically.
- Disorganised and may find it difficult completing projects such as homework – output increases when allowed to use technology, which should be an appropriate strategy with IT training and support.

This information is advisory only – dyslexia or dyslexic tendencies should only be formally diagnosed by an educational psychologist, specialist teacher, paediatrician or other suitably trained professional.

Dyscalculia

Dyscalculia is regarded as a specific learning difficulty relating to understanding and writing numbers, including arithmetic. Dyscalculia has been described as dyslexia for numbers.

The American Psychiatric Association (2013) describes dyscalculia as a specific learning disorder that is characterised by difficulties learning basic arithmetic facts, processing numbers and performing accurate and fluent calculations. These difficulties must be quantifiably below what is expected for an individual's chronological age, and must not be caused by more significant intellectual impairments.

Dyscalculia, as with other neuro-diversities, may be present as a standalone issue, or with overlapping issues as highlighted in Figure 2.2.

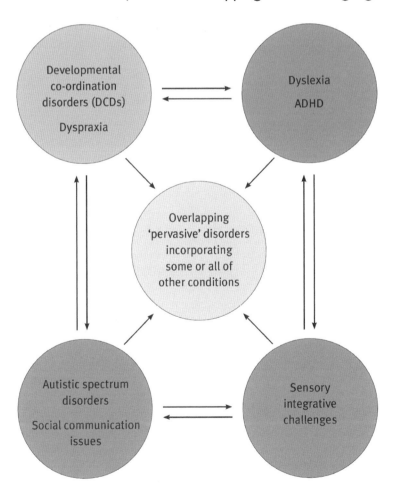

Figure 2.2   Issues that may coexist with developmental coordination disorder

Educational psychologists are best placed to provide assessment and helpful recommendations for young people with number difficulties. Specialist teachers are well placed to provide support for children with dyscalculia.

Attention deficit hyperactivity disorder

This can be an overlapping condition with developmental coordination disorder (DCD). Information in this section is taken from the Centers for Disease Control and Prevention website – see 'References' section). This information is advisory only, and this condition should only be formally diagnosed by a paediatrician or allied specialist, such as an educational psychologist.

For an appropriate diagnosis of attention deficit hyperactivity disorder (ADHD) some of the child's symptoms should be present before they reach the age of 7 and be identifiable in more than one setting. There should be clear evidence of an adverse effect on the child's schoolwork, social settings and everyday tasks. The indicators of ADHD in a child are listed below.

Inattention
Six or more of the symptoms indicated below need to be present for at least six months, causing disruptive and inappropriate behaviour (bearing in mind the child's age).

- The child has difficulty in attending to detail and makes careless mistakes in schoolwork and allied activities.
- They are easily distracted: they pay too much attention to what is going on around them at the expense of concentrating on the activity in hand.
- They find it hard to maintain focus on tasks, and their interest jumps around from one play activity to another.
- They do not appear to listen or hear when spoken to directly.
- They do not follow instructions and fail to finish their homework or tasks even though they have understood the instructions.
- Organising projects and activities is challenging for the child.
- They dislike and will avoid extended projects in school or homework.
- Equipment such as books, pens or toys is constantly lost or 'misplaced' by the child.
- They can be forgetful in personal care and general life skills.

Hyperactivity

Six or more symptoms of hyperactivity and impulsivity need to be present for at least six months, causing disruptive and inappropriate behaviour (bearing in mind the child's age).

- The child often fidgets and fiddles with hands and objects, squirms and shifts in their seat. See details on the Moro and spinal Galant reflexes in Chapter 7.
- They are often up and down from the seat when expected to sit – for example, during meal times.
- They are often running about when and where it is not appropriate.
- They have difficulty playing with or enjoying fun/leisure activities quietly.
- They are often 'on the go' as though being driven by a motor.
- They may talk excessively.

Impulsivity

- The child regularly blurts out answers before questions have been completed.
- They often have trouble taking turns.
- They interrupt others on a regular basis.

These children may be experiencing heightened stress levels as a result of a poorly integrated Moro or 'startle' reflex. This can keep them in a heightened 'flight, fight or fear' mode – see information on sensory integration (Chapter 3) and the Moro reflex (Chapter 7). Some of the above symptoms may be seen in children with a sensory integrative dysfunction, and a sensory profile should be undertaken by a suitably qualified practitioner.

The National Institute for Health Excellence (NICE) details guidance on diagnosis and advances in treatment for young people and adults with ADD and or ADHD. See their website: nice.org.uk

Autistic spectrum disorders

Children whose challenges fall within the autistic spectrum are very individual, but they may experience what is called a 'Triad of Impairment' (Wing, 2003) that defines their overall condition.

1. **Communication challenges**
   - Speech, communication and language difficulties.
   - A lack of intonation in speech.
   - Limited gestures such as pointing.
   - Facial expressions and own body language may be minimal, and the child may not be able to pick up these cues from those around them.

2. **Socialisation**
   - Difficulties in engaging with and making social relationships with their peers.
   - May have poor social timing and find interaction difficult.
   - Lack empathy and awareness of the emotional and physical needs of others.
   - May not have an automatic sense of their own body position in space and stand too close or too far away from others.
   - There may be a rejection of or resistance to normal body contact because of touch sensitivity, for example, when being greeted or hugged.
   - Do not make appropriate eye contact, or eye contact may be very limited.

3. **Theory of mind**
   - Rigidity and lack of flexibility of thought processes.
   - Resistant to change, and find transitions from one situation to another difficult.
   - Lack of understanding of a situation, particularly if new.
   - Obsessional and ritualistic behaviour.
   - Preference for engaging in activities, videos and games they feel 'safe' with and which a younger child would normally engage in.

Children with autism may also have a range of sensory challenges – for example, a heightened sensitivity to:

■ Touch
■ Sound
■ Vision
■ Smell and taste.

Alternatively, they may have a reduced registration or awareness of pain or discomfort. They may also have a limited sense of their own body and limb scheme in space (proprioception). There may be overlapping dyslexic or dyspraxic tendencies in the child with an autistic spectrum disorder. Clusters of retained primitive 'baby' reflexes may also be observed adversely affecting the child's motor coordination (see the section on reflexes in Chapter 7).

The advice of professionals, including an occupational therapist with experience in sensory integrative and processing disorders, can provide a fuller understanding of the issues raised and practical strategies to support this condition, particularly in relation to schooling.

Developmental language disorder

Developmental language disorder (previously known as specific language impairment) is a persistent type of speech, language and communication need that cannot be related to an obvious cause.

DLD may be identified in children when their development of talking:

- Falls behind others of the same age
- Interferes in everyday life, including school achievement
- Is not due to hearing loss, physical abnormality, acquired brain damage or lack of experience
- Is not part of a general delay in development which affects all other skills.

Speech and language therapy is an essential service for young people with communication difficulties. This area should be addressed as soon as possible, as the ability to communicate is essential for social relationships, activities of daily living and for learning new skills.

Your GP or paediatrician can make a referral to see a speech and language therapist, providing the points above are identified (see Royal College of Speech and Language Therapists in the 'Professional organisations' section).

Associated challenges: self-esteem issues

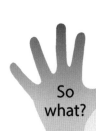

So what: issues and challenges

◆ Children with DCD, including dyspraxia, have average or above average intelligence, but can experience a loss of personal self-esteem for a variety of reasons.

◆ There may be a mismatch between the child's innate intelligence and their reduced functional performance because of sensory and motor learning challenges.

◆ This may result from the underlying developmental immaturity which has not been identified and is therefore poorly understood by the child and those in daily contact with them.

◆ Avoidance strategies for tasks and activities which the child finds difficult can start to emerge even before they are established in school. They have a sense that they are struggling but do not understand why. As the child is intelligent they 'know' there is something wrong.

◆ A poor sense of self-esteem is also common in children with an overlapping profile of dyspraxia/dyslexia and is compounded by peers, who can be quick to recognise that the child is struggling in written work, games and PE. They can then feel isolated and alone, particularly in a competitive environment.

◆ It is not uncommon for these intelligent children to be placed in low achieving groups in class, as the specific issues may not be recognised or appropriate practical support and strategies provided to optimise their ability.

◆ The child may see themselves as 'stupid', 'useless', state that the work is 'boring', and become oppositional and reluctant to engage in activities that have not previously been successful for them.

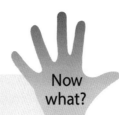

Now what?

Now what: practical strategies and ideas

- Additional support and monitoring from the class teacher, providing positive feedback for the effort made by the child, as opposed to purely the end product in schoolwork.

- Should the child continue to struggle and self-esteem be adversely affected, advice should be sought from external agencies to provide understanding and strategies, and to evaluate any underlying sensory motor challenges.

- An occupational therapist with a working knowledge of sensory integration can provide a comprehensive assessment of the child's strengths and challenges, incorporating clinical observations and standardised tests. Strategies and advice can then be integrated into the school day and home life.

- The advice of an educational psychologist can also be extremely valuable to ascertain the child's innate cognitive skills as well as their physical output. Any hidden agendas such as dyslexia or dyslexic tendencies can then be identified to assist the child and their mentors.

- 'Gentle teaching' – initiated by Dan Hobbs in America to support individuals with challenging behaviour – sets out the following prerequisites for success in supporting children and young people with additional needs. Activities and engagement for children with learning difficulties should be:

    (a) Safe
    (b) Fair
    (c) Dignifying to the child
    (d) The 'just right' challenge
    (e) Fun.

- Some differentiation in PE and games may be required, but should be provided in such a way that the child with dyspraxia does not feel set apart.

- Additional practice of specific therapy exercises can be incorporated, particularly for the younger primary age child. The Institute for Neuro-Physiological Psychology can recommend practitioners undertaking this work (see INPP in the 'Professional organisations' section).

- Peer pairing may be of value and also allocating a key member of staff whom the child can specifically refer to for day-to-day issues of organisation, time frames, planning, sequencing and carrying out projects.

- Set functional achievable goals with the child, teacher and parent to enable the child to feel supported and more in control.

- Realistic praise and positive reinforcement will result in a happier and less stressed child; planning and identifying specific issues once a term will also assist.

- There are a considerable number of providers of material to support self-esteem issues (see Speechmark and Winslow in the 'Resources' section of this book).

Associated challenges: depression/ mood-related disorders

Mental health issues are regrettably the biggest secondary factor for young people with neuro-diversities, including developmental coordination disorder. However, this can be alleviated with timely assessment and support from health and education professionals, in conjunction with young people and their families.

Children who are withdrawn, the class clown, or have persistent difficulties with friendships should be screened for undiagnosed neuro-diversity as well as referral to mental health support services.

Children with high levels of anxiety and reduced self-esteem are at risk from developing clinical depression. If this occurs, it is imperative that the child has ongoing support from their GP and the Child Adolescent Mental Health Service (CAHMS). When psychological aspects are appropriately supported, the child can actively engage and participate in occupational therapy and school, including the ability to take on board new ideas and try out new strategies.

Communication between physical, mental health and education professionals is the key to holistic and timely support for the child. It often comes down to parents and caregivers to facilitate or prompt this communication, given the requirement for informed consent.

Mind is a well-established charity, committed to providing information and support, and, ultimately, to help people improve and maintain their mental health. It has some excellent online resources and a helpline, which provides support for young people and their families living with mental health difficulties (see Mind in the 'Professional organisations' section).

Chapter 3

Sensory integration

Overview

Sensory integration is the ability to take in, process and organise all the information around us through our different senses in order to respond and act appropriately within our environment.

- This surrounding sensory information must be filtered, organised, integrated and then modulated appropriately for successful 'sensory integration' to take place.
- Individuals with a sensory integrative dysfunction and sensory processing difficulties may not be able to process external stimuli in an integrated way, and as a result their responses may not be appropriate to a given situation.
- If these systems are over- or under-responsive, or fluctuate in their functioning, there can be an altered perception in the individual of what is going on, not only around them but also within their own body, which may then result in an inappropriate response or reaction.
- Children with developmental coordination disorder (DCD) can be both under-responsive and over-responsive even within one sensory system. They can take longer to register something but when they do, they can quickly be overwhelmed by it and not have the ability to respond or adjust to the stimuli easily.
- Sensory integrative dysfunction has an adverse effect on everyday life. A child's responses may sometimes be seen as an emotional or behavioural issue as opposed to what is, in reality, a physiological one. If unrecognised, genuine emotional and behavioural difficulties may accumulate.

- There are several different senses (sensory systems) through which we process information:

    1. Vestibular (static and moving balance/orientation)
    2. Tactile (touch)
    3. Proprioceptive (body scheme and position awareness)
    4. Visual (looking and seeing)
    5. Auditory (hearing)
    6. Olfactory and gustatory (smell and taste).

Vestibular/balance system (see full description later in chapter)

- If the child's vestibular system is over-reactive, they may be very sensitive to movement, avoid unnecessary movement and be reluctant to engage in activities which involve height or very active movement such as climbing. The child may experience car sickness and feel dizzy easily. Their static and moving balance is likely to be poor, and they may have a poor sense of orientation in space.

- Alternatively, if the child's vestibular system is under-reactive and slow to respond to movement input, the child may be a movement seeker and be 'on the go' much of the time – swinging, spinning, jumping, running and generally seeking movement in a desire to 'prime' this system and gain the level of stimulation that they need to feel 'integrated' – but usually in a manner over and above the level for their age. The younger child may become very agile and adept at climbing onto any surface they can find!

Touch (see full description later in chapter)

- A child may register touch in an under reactive way as a result of poor registration through their tactile systems. This can make manipulation and manual dexterity difficult, and the child may also have a reduced sense of their own body scheme, making the organisation and planning of movement difficult. They may be messy eaters as they are unaware of where the food is in their mouths due to reduced sensory awareness. Children with a reduced touch sensitivity may also not be aware when they have hurt themselves, and may appear very stoic in the face of an injury due to their lack of registration of pain or discomfort.

■ Alternatively, many children with sensory integrative dysfunction may have a high level of sensitivity to touch and find handling, touching and the textures of clothes extremely uncomfortable. These children may well overreact to contact with others, resulting in an overt and inappropriate response. They find life in general more threatening and may lose focus or concentration on their schoolwork because of their sensitivity. Hypersensitivity to touch is common in children with autistic spectrum disorders. A child with autism may have a sensory integrative disorder, but a child with sensory integrative dysfunction does not necessarily have autistic tendencies. Children with a heightened awareness of touch may seek contact but on their own terms, and they may 'mouth' and chew things, which is normal in a young child but sometimes inappropriate in an older one.

Body awareness/proprioception (see full description later in chapter)

■ The child with dyspraxia, as mentioned, may have a poor sense of their own body scheme and spatial awareness. There is a tendency to be accident prone, heavy footed (and handed), bump into things, and be unaware of the force they are using in everyday tasks.

Looking and seeing

■ Although a child with dyspraxia may have reasonable vision, the organisation of visual information, its throughput and response may be a little slower – especially for visual perceptual tasks. It is also not uncommon to observe difficulties in the child's ability to fix their eyes on a moving object and visually track it in the horizontal or vertical plane. Their eyes may blink or 'jump' at the body midline due to a lack of integration of both sides of the body. Activities such as copying from the board, locating their vision from board to desk, and far and near focus difficulties may adversely affect their schoolwork. Blurring may occur during and following movement. Ball games and allied activities will be difficult as a result. (See the section on vision and eye movement control in Chapter 4.)

Hearing

■ Chronic ear infections may affect the child's ability to hear distinctly, and this in turn will affect speech output. Despite a successful hearing test, very high and low sounds may be missed. The child with dyspraxia may hear but be unable to process the sounds and lose focus. A busy, noisy environment may cause 'sensory' overload, which in turn causes reduced attention and concentration. They may also take longer to process auditory information and require extra time to take information in and respond accordingly.

Taste and smell

■ These senses are very closely linked. Food may not taste very exciting if the child has a blocked nose and sinus problems, resulting in disinterest in eating. Alternatively, many children with sensory integration challenges have a heightened sense of taste and smell, resulting in a refusal to eat many foods. These children may have a strong 'gag' reflex and a tendency to choke and cough up food, especially if sensitive to certain textured and 'lumpy' food.

A multi-sensory approach to learning

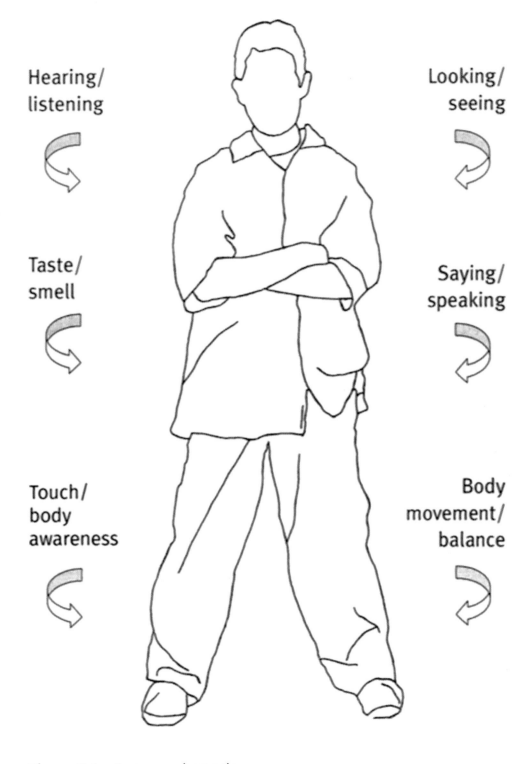

Hearing/
listening

Looking/
seeing

Taste/
smell

Saying/
speaking

Touch/
body
awareness

Body
movement/
balance

Figure 3.1   Sensory channels

Learning acquisition – sensory processing

As mentioned, the acquisition of information about ourselves and from the environment around us comes via a whole range of senses, as illustrated in Figure 3.1. This information has to be received, processed, filtered and organised in order for each individual to give an appropriate motor response to any given input. For some children with a developmental coordination disorder or dyspraxia, one or more of these systems may not be functioning at an optimal level. It is therefore vital that other learning methods are incorporated through a multi-sensory approach, especially in the early years, to allow the child to function comfortably and make sense of the information coming in from their environment. From birth babies and children acquire and hone skills which progress from a combination of apparently random, reactive or reflexive involuntary movements to organised, refined and controlled motor output as their systems mature.

Particularly in a primary school situation, desks and tables need to face the focus of teaching to allow both the visual and auditory learning pathways to work together in order to give each child the best chance to consolidate their learning. The child is also able to pick up the teacher's 'body language' and facial expressions, giving them additional learning cues. A twenty-year study at Nottingham Trent University concluded that pupils sitting in rows facing the teacher learn far more than those sitting in groups where some have their backs to the teacher (Hastings & Chantrey Wood, 2002). Professor Nigel Hastings and his colleague, Karen Chantrey Wood, reported that up to 50 per cent of a child's learning can be adversely affected when placed in a group with their back to the teacher, particularly in the case of children who are easily distracted. In their view, although sitting in rows may not necessarily be better than sitting around tables, traditional seating with all the children facing the teacher is far better for most lessons. Some children may be primarily 'visual' rather than 'auditory' learners, so sitting facing the teacher and the focus of teaching is particularly important for them. Dyspraxic children also require longer quiet periods to allow consolidation of information.

Every preschool child should be given the maximum opportunity to learn through both child- and adult-directed activities incorporating movement, exploration and games in the early years. This allows adequate sensory/motor integration in preparation for school learning. Findings indicate that if a child has not had sufficient opportunity for play experiences, they will be ill-equipped for academic learning, and indeed introducing formal learning from the age of 3 or 4 could be retrogressive for them as they are not developmentally equipped for the demands placed on them. Nevertheless, there are some children with motor learning difficulties who will continue to experience challenges in regard to physical output and require additional practical support and strategies.

The vestibular (balance) system

What? ## What: definition and meaning

- The vestibular system is based within the inner ear in the brain and is interdependent with all the other body systems, including the proprioceptive and tactile (touch) systems.

- The fluid within the inner ear apparatus (semi-circular canals) contains thousands of tiny hairs, which register and react to different positions of the head, neck and body.

- Messages are then sent to different parts of the body to enable the child to make an 'adaptive' movement response and to interact appropriately with their environment.

- The vestibular system may be over-sensitive to movement in some children with dyspraxia, resulting in fear of movement in sport and general physical activities, particularly where balance is integral to the activity.

- Alternatively, the vestibular system may be under-reactive, and the child may be constantly movement seeking and 'on the go' in an unconscious effort to stimulate and mature this system.

The vestibular system can influence:

- Moving and static (standing) balance skills.
- Functional eye movements and the ability to fix on and follow moving objects in different planes, as well as to move the eyes in a more rapid movement from one place to another.
- Posture and level of muscle tone, which may be low, high or within a normal range.
- Physical and spatial orientation in relation to the environment.
- Integrating both sides of the body together – see the section on bilateral integration in Chapter 6.
- The child's level of focus and ability to attend.

A story is told of a team of astronauts working in space. When temporarily placed in zero gravity with a resulting loss of spatial orientation, they began 'mirror' writing when recording information.

When reorientated to gravity, normal writing patterns resumed, indicating that the disruption of the underlying balance systems can impact on writing and recording output. Mirror writing may be observed in very young children and also those with dyslexic tendencies over the age of 7 or 8. This may indicate that immature or damaged balance systems have a role to play in some handwriting challenges. However, this is only one possible underlying contributor to a dyslexic and/or dyspraxic profile; other contributory factors may have a visual or auditory origin, or be a result of motor or general learning difficulties.

So what: issues and challenges

So what?

◆ The vestibular system may be within the norm, but in some children with dyspraxia it is under-reactive or over-reactive.

◆ If under-reactive, the child is likely to be excessively movement seeking, finding it difficult to sit still for extended periods – they need to jump, run, bundle, roll and be generally 'on the go'. As they get older they may seek activities that offer enhanced speed and extreme movement, and the child may appear relatively fearless in their pursuit of movement.

◆ Alternatively, the child with an over-reactive or sensitive vestibular system may appear timid, fearful of movement and very wary of anything that challenges their balance mechanisms, even to the extent of experiencing anxiety when going down stairs, and especially on escalators, due to a lack of postural and balance control.

◆ Moving and static (standing) balance may be affected. The child may have difficulty in balancing on one leg, as, for example, when getting dressed. They may have difficulty keeping their balance on PE equipment and be reluctant to engage in play activities involving climbing and walking along kerbs or low walls.

◆ Reading may be adversely affected as the child cannot maintain smooth visual tracking along the line on the page. They may lose their place when looking up at the board and back to their work and/or experience blurring. It therefore takes longer to accommodate their vision when looking from one point to another and to get information down on paper within normal time frames.

◆ The child may have difficulty watching and visually tracking a moving object such as a ball to catch it or hit it with a bat, and may easily become car sick due to the higher level of visual activity when travelling by car or other transport.

◆ The child may have rather 'floppy' low muscle tone affecting their exercise tolerance. The ability to maintain an upright posture at the table for extended periods will be compromised, they will tire more easily in class than their peers and may become fidgety.

◆ The child's 'saving' reactions may be weak – that is, the ability to automatically put their arms out in front of them for protection if they fall, causing them to fall more heavily with increased risk of injury.

◆ The child may lack the ability to deal with all the extraneous visual and auditory stimuli in class

◆ The child's ability to coordinate both sides of the body for use (bilateral integration) and/or to work both sides of the body together for reciprocal (cross-pattern) movements may be limited.

◆ The child may shift to one side in their chair to avoid working across their body midline when writing across the page, due again to a lack of integration between two sides of the body.

◆ Sequencing of instructions and activities may be difficult, and the child's confidence, attention and concentration can then be affected. The child who struggles to organise both themselves and their work in class, will feel as though they are always a 'step behind' their colleagues.

◆ Frequently children with vestibular dysfunction lack a strong sense of self.

Now what?

Now what: practical strategies and ideas

● Movement opportunities should be provided where possible, prior to schoolwork for the younger child. Linear movement such as swinging and running and also slow rotation movements are soothing, and can provide input to both an under-reactive and over-reactive vestibular system, enabling the child to attend and focus in their work. Note: Never continue to swing or spin a child after they ask you to stop. At that point, they have had enough stimulation.

- Provide the child with supportive seating with the desk at elbow height, knees at 90 degrees and feet firmly on the floor for stability.

- An angled board, desk or folder is recommended to maintain good posture and head position.

- Differentiation for recording of information may be required by the teacher. Ensure the child faces the information source in class and is given additional time to record written information. Provide copies of notes as appropriate.

- Ensure the child does not feel overly pressured and that instructions are clearly reinforced in a multi-sensory way (spoken, demonstrated and/or written).

- Allow movement or short respite breaks to ease any discomfort for children with weaker or lower muscle tone and be aware that they may tire more easily.

- Give time for practical organisation of materials.

- Encourage a dominant hand by placing work to the dominant side – this will also stop the child twisting and turning in their seat as a result of any difficulty in working across their body midline.

- Exercises to enhance muscle tone can be advised upon by a physiotherapist or occupational therapist as part of an overall functional assessment.

- A child may have difficulties with visual tracking despite a positive optician's eye test report. Advice should be sought from an optometrist on functional vision (see British Association of Behavioural Optometrists (BABO) in the 'Professional organisations' section); this can then be incorporated into the child's school and home setting.

- Give every opportunity to enhance balance at the 'just right' level to maintain confidence and self-esteem. Offer positive feedback for effort made as opposed to the end result where the activity is challenging.

- Plan ahead the night before for suitable books; provide a 'see through' pencil case, ensuring that the contents are maintained in working order.
- Colour code both timetable and subject books; where a laptop is used, provide a copy of an updated timetable as a screen saver or easily accessible document on work/home book.
- Allow some differentiation in PE and games to compensate for poor static or dynamic balance while ensuring that the child does not feel set apart from their peers.
- Encourage integrating, cross-pattern exercises in PE. Ideally seek exercises from a physiotherapist or occupational therapist trained in sensory integration.
- Allow the child who has identifiable fears to practise activities in their own time and again at the 'just right' level of challenge. Their systems may not be physiologically altered but confidence can be enhanced, resulting in an effective improvement.

The tactile (touch awareness) system

What: definition and meaning

What?

- Our touch system consists of two main parts: one part responds to lighter touch and the other to deep or firm touch pressure. The balance in these two systems helps us to recognise the difference between touch that is helpful or harmful – for example, when handling sharp, hot or cold objects.
- An integrated touch system allows the child to focus their attention and influences body awareness and motor planning. It also allows them to interact with and engage with the environment effectively.
- Many children with dyspraxia can experience a lack of 'balance' in this vital system of touch, and the resulting sensory information they receive can adversely affect their ability to function to their best level – as, for example, in overall coordination for fine and large motor skills.
- As the touch system is closely connected with the body awareness and balance systems, strategies are likely to overlap.

So what: issues and challenges

So what?

For children with hypersensitive touch systems the following may occur:

◆ The child may find physical contact of any sort unpleasant. They can overreact to nudging, pushing or people standing close to them. They may shrug and move away when anyone attempts to make contact with them, or in the case of a child with extreme touch sensitivity, react in an aggressive manner when contact is made with those around them. (This and allied sensory processing issues (see below) can be common in children with autistic spectrum disorders as well as in those with dyspraxia.)

◆ The child may find it hard to sit still or focus on what is going on around them, as they have a heightened registration of discomfort from clothes textures and other environmental contact.

◆ The child may find it difficult to sit comfortably on a hard floor or surface and have trouble getting comfortable and off to sleep at night when their bedding is not 'just right'.

◆ They may be more sensitive to pain and cry easily as injury and discomfort are registered at a much higher level.

◆ The child may be intolerant of having hair washed, teeth cleaned or nails cut.

◆ The child may be more emotional as a result of the above and express anger or anxiety easily. Their systems appear in 'flight or fight' mode, and indeed a poorly integrated Moro reflex may be present which puts the child into a heightened state of awareness, affecting and alerting sensory systems such as vision and hearing (see Chapter 7).

◆ The child may seek out touch contact by putting objects to their mouth (normal in a very young child) and generally being 'touchy feely', but on their own terms and not always appropriately, as this is a less threatening way of receiving the stimulus their body needs.

For children with an under-reactive touch system the following may occur:

◆ Play activities may be of less interest as touch feedback is poor.

◆ Tasks requiring manipulation, such as picking up fine objects, doing up buttons and shoelaces, and handwriting, will be difficult due to a lack of sensitivity and feedback in the hands and fingers.

◆ The child's sense of their own body scheme may be weak. Clothes may be untidy, not tucked in or positioned correctly, not through choice but as a consequence of a general lack of awareness/feedback.

◆ The child may not register when they have hurt themselves – for example, if they have rubbed a blister on the back of their heel or cut themselves. They tend to be the 'long suffering' or stoic child who puts up with a lot of discomfort due to the reduced feedback and perception of discomfort through their touch systems.

◆ The child may not know the force they are using when gripping and handling objects and may break objects easily (also as a result of a lack of proprioceptive (body and limb position) awareness). This can affect motor planning and organisation for activities.

Now what: practical strategies and ideas

Now what?

Strategies for the child with heightened tactile registration:

● Assist the older child to find their own strategies by explaining that they feel touch and pain discomfort more easily than others – particularly if it is unexpected – and therefore need to be aware of this when in crowds, or involved in contact sports and school activities. This will avoid an overreaction on the child's part, as they are more prepared.

● Allow the child additional space where possible in the class setting and around mealtimes – for example, when in a queue.

● When sitting for extended periods on the floor, they may need a small mat or be allowed movement opportunities to ease physical discomfort.

● Ensure that if sensitive to small injuries, these are handled with the minimum of fuss; monitor contact sports/PE to minimise unnecessary problems.

● Ensure where possible that the child is supported in a calm manner; avoid raised voices and minimise noise in a busy situation as this can relieve tension and soothe heightened touch systems.

● At home, ensure that any scratchy clothing labels are removed, use natural materials for clothing where possible, avoid tight belts or buttoning, and provide socks which are heelless.

● Baths may be less painful than showers. In the bath, slowly and gently rub or massage the head using moderate, comforting pressure prior to hair washing. Dry with a towel after bath. Prior to nail cutting, gently squeeze nails and tips of fingers. Encourage the child to massage gums with a cloth using their index finger before (and after) teeth cleaning to ease discomfort.

● Techniques such as brushing the skin and providing therapeutic 'proprioceptive' input can assist in integrating the touch sensitive system – under the direction of an occupational therapist trained in sensory integration. This treatment requires commitment and time on the part of both the parent and the child, but can have successful outcomes in some individuals.

Strategies for the child with poor touch registration and discrimination:

- Prior to a tabletop activity provide movement opportunities for the child to alert the nervous system. Try 'star jumps', running on the spot, stretching out and shaking arms and hands, wriggling fingers.

- Place extra paper under the child's written work to take pressure off the pen. Allow short breaks to ease hand discomfort due to additional pressure in hand and fingers.

- Ensure that games and activities for younger children have a variety of textures and materials to ensure interest and engagement. Use activities with a visual interest as a compensatory mechanism.

- Monitor the child for any injury sustained such as bruising and blisters which may not have been registered by them.

- Where necessary provide adapted clothing such as Velcro instead of laces. Replace existing buttons with textured larger ones for the younger child.

- Provide multi-sensory games such as Twister and the Body Game to integrate body awareness and touch systems.

- Practise action games and rhymes such as Head, Shoulders, Knees and Toes and Simon Says – at a slower rate for younger children – which allow the child to plan and organise their movements.

- It may be necessary to have a full sensory profile undertaken under the remit of an occupational therapist and in tandem with other screening tests in order to evaluate a child's strengths and challenges. The child can then be better supported at school and home with a fuller understanding of their sensory needs.

The proprioceptive (body position awareness) system

What: definition and meaning

What?

This is a sensory system which should automatically inform us of where our body and limb position is in space when outside our field of vision. It is one of the key areas inherent to dyspraxia. Receptors in our joints and muscles should automatically provide this feedback and allow 'motor' planning of movement without any real conscious awareness once skills are acquired.

This sensory system can often be under-reactive in children with DCD/dyspraxia, resulting in a reduced sense of body and limb position in space in relation to the environment. This can have an adverse impact both on movement and on everyday activities.

Most people can recall their first driving lesson – an exciting but stressful experience. Every action needs to be thought about – steering wheel, clutch, brake, accelerator, mirror, handbrake – even before turning the engine on to move forward. Only after careful planning and multi-tasking in the correct sequence can we think about driving the car. With practice driving finally becomes automatic, and we undertake a sequence of moves without constant cognitive monitoring.

Children with a reduced sense of their own body scheme and limb position awareness often remain at the stage where every movement must be cognitively planned, nothing is automatic, and they have to consciously visually monitor and think about their movements, often at the expense of the activity in hand, for example handwriting formation.

The proprioceptive system is very rarely over-responsive.

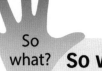

So what: issues and challenges

♦ A child with this challenge is experiencing one of the key underlying issues in dyspraxia. Reduced proprioception can result in ongoing difficulties in the planning and organisation of movements, making daily routines much harder and more tiring for them. It can affect all large and fine motor skills, including handwriting.

♦ The child may have difficulty in positioning their body spatially for sitting, standing, getting on and off, over and around or through equipment, or just moving about a room. As a result they may be reluctant to engage in many physical activities.

♦ A child with reduced proprioception may be 'movement seeking' and unable to sit still for long, and they need to move and fidget to remain sufficiently alert in class. This is also common in children with an under-reactive vestibular system.

♦ The child may be accident prone with a tendency to trip over their own feet, bump into objects, lack awareness of the force they are using, be heavy handed and footed. When jumping they lack spring and the ability to land lightly.

♦ Physical activity is more tiring for them as they may also have poorer muscle tone and postural strength. A child with low proprioception or kinaesthetic awareness may be perceived as lazy and slow, whereas in reality they are often innately intelligent but lack the motor skills and confidence to reflect this.

♦ The child may take longer to get dressed, dress untidily and be unaware of clothes being inside out and poorly tucked in. The child may be a 'messy' eater and generally poorly organised.

♦ In tandem with poor touch registration, the child may not always register pain and will tolerate discomfort when hurt or injured. They appear stoic and uncomplaining.

♦ Alternatively, some children with reduced body awareness find that their other sensory systems such as touch, hearing and vision are heightened, causing distractibility and loss of focus.

♦ They fidget to 'alert' this under-reactive sensory system and find it hard to sit still, or alternatively have loss of focus when sitting for extended periods and 'tune out'.

- They may lack awareness of the general force they are using in contact sports, hugging and playing with others. They may break toys and equipment without meaning to and may hurt others unwittingly.
- Excessive pressure on their pen, breaking nibs, also causes the child to complain of their hand tiring after writing for a relatively short period as they cannot monitor feedback from the pressure they are exerting; they may keep stopping to shake their writing hand.
- Spatial awareness when recording information on paper may be weak. Writing may be messy and poorly coordinated, as with general manual dexterity. Laces are often loose due to difficulty in manipulation.
- A lack of self-confidence and self-esteem may be observed.

Now what: practical strategies and ideas

Now what?

- Provide the child with warm-up exercises prior to focused work. Gentle push or pull (resisted) activities can alert the proprioceptive system and 'wake' the child up.
- The child should face the focus of teaching.
- Ensure that the child's sitting is symmetrical and well supported, with feet firmly on floor and body correctly positioned to gain feedback through their body.
- Use of a 'Move 'n' Sit' (see Back in Action in the 'Resources' section) or other design of angled cushion to allow the child 'contained' movement at the desk can be helpful for children who need to fidget to keep alert.
- Allow the child movement opportunities such as handing out books at regular intervals in class.
- Provide the child with an angled board, folder or worktop to assist them to maintain an upright position at the desk and avoid strain on back and shoulders. Laptops should also be angled.
- The teacher should provide extra paper under written work to ease pressure on the hand and pen.
- Allow the child extra time for copying tasks, especially when working from a board.

- Provide pens and pencils with integral grips to ease discomfort and provide tactile (touch) feedback. Advice from an occupational therapist can assist in this and other related areas of function.

- Provide the child with templates, graph paper and visual cues where appropriate to assist spatial presentation on paper.

- Keyboard training with the use of a laptop may be appropriate to ease pressure on the hand when writing, particularly prior to secondary stage, and can then be integrated into the school lessons and ultimately used for tests and examinations.

- Allow the child some differentiation for sports, PE and games in general in order for them to succeed and maintain their confidence and self-esteem.

- Staff should give positive feedback for the effort made by the child as opposed to the final result during activities that are challenging.

Chapter 4

Eye and hand skills

Visual motor integration

There is a strong overlap between the sections on visual motor integration and handwriting as the two areas are interdependent.

What?

What: definition and meaning

- It is the ability to receive, process and interpret visual information (visual perception) and then translate it with a motor action (physical movement) onto paper with the use of adequate hand and finger control. This is important for all activities involving vision and movement, including writing, drawing and mark-making on paper. The use of technology such as a tablet or computer also requires these skills.
- It is a primary requisite for schooling.
- Visual motor integration requires, among other skills, reasonable eye function, postural stability and upper limb motor control, and visual spatial ability as well as cognitive skills.
- Difficulties integrating visual information with the motor output may be in the visual interpretation of the recorded forms (visual perception), or alternatively in the physical ability to reproduce the perceived information.
- Many children with dyspraxia have a mismatch between their cognitive, or thinking skills and their exhibited motor ability – the latter being the main difficulty.

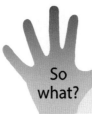

So what?

So what: issues and challenges

♦ Difficulty with handwriting and recording of tasks although verbally able.

♦ Poor control of pen. Immature fixed pen grip as in a palmar grasp, with the thumb lapped across the pen, or a static as opposed to dynamic 'tripod' (three-fingered grip).

♦ Whole arm movements may occur, making output more tiring than for the child's peers when recording information due to the lack of refinement of pen control.

♦ May press too hard on paper or pressure fluctuates on paper, which is more effortful.

♦ When pen or pencil pressure fluctuates on paper, it can result in different densities of text, making it harder to read.

♦ The child may tend to 'pen push', which may be due to the retained presence of an asymmetrical tonic neck reflex. An involuntary extension movement of the arm may be elicited by the child turning their head to look at their writing hand. (This movement can be clearly seen in very young babies – see the section on asymmetrical tonic neck reflex in Chapter 7 for further information.)

♦ When recording information, the child may lean to one side to avoid writing across their body midline due to poor integration of both sides of the body, or alternatively shift their whole body to one side, incurring more effort for them than for their peers.

♦ The child may not be able to draw intersecting lines past the midline if they lack integration enables each side of the child's body to do things simultaneously. An example of this is one hand holding the paper and the other using the pen.

♦ Children who lack integration of both sides of the body (see the bilateral integration section in Chapter 6) may also have difficulty copying from notes at the side of their desk as their eyes fail to work smoothly in the horizontal plane – a midline blink of the eyes may be noted if they are asked to fix on and watch a moving object with their eyes in the horizontal position.

♦ The child may slump over the desk or head prop on one hand (due to poor core stability, weak tummy and back muscles); the distance between hand and eye then becomes too short to sustain consistent eye muscle contraction, which can cause eyestrain (the distance should be a forearm length between eyes and paper).

◆ The child may not sit correctly on their chair due to a reduced sense of their body position awareness in space, and may need to be reminded to place themselves and the chair in the correct position (see proprioception section in Chapter 3).

◆ Postural stability at shoulders and trunk and level of muscle tone may also be weak, making it hard for the child to maintain an upright position. Core stability is important for sustained sitting on a classroom chair.

◆ Poor representation or orientation of one shape to another (spatial orientation) or ability to maintain line position may be noted.

◆ Loss of orientation when changing direction when drawing angled shapes may be noted (this can indicate dyslexic tendencies if occurring consistently in children above 7 or 8 years of age).

◆ Fidgeting and the inability to sit for extended periods may be noted (possibly due to mechanical discomfort as a result of presence of the symmetrical and/or asymmetrical tonic neck reflex).

◆ Fidgeting may also occur as a result of the need for the child to maintain alertness due to an under-reactive body position awareness (proprioceptive) system.

◆ Difficulty may be experienced with copying work, graphics and drawing tasks, but particularly copying from the board, use of scissors, building models, apparatus work.

◆ Underlying visual perceptual challenges may be a major part of the child's difficulties.

Now what: practical strategies and ideas

Now what?

● The teacher should ensure that the child faces the focus of the teaching and the interactive board or chalkboard when copying and drawing to minimise the effect of whole body movement.

● A formal check of functional vision (see BABO in the 'Professional organisations' section) is advised to exclude any concerns within this remit.

- Improve pen control by using activities such as peg games to build up a pincer grip between index finger and thumb, and to help the child to isolate finger and thumb movements. A dynamic tripod grip should be encouraged when using a pen, pencil or stylus.

- An occupational therapist can provide a range of standardised and non-standardised tests to ascertain the main underlying contributors to the child's difficulties.

- Exercises can be provided to work on the child's whole shoulder and arm patterns and integration of both sides of the body under the direction of an occupational therapist (reflex inhibition exercises).

- The child's forearm should be supported on an angled board, folder or desk, allowing the hand to be placed correctly with the wrist slightly extended. This allows the fingers and thumb to fall into a natural pincer grip on the pen, which facilitates the fluid movement needed for cursive writing.

- An angled writing surface will also limit the need for head propping and 'slumping' at the desk and ease back and neck tension.

- The child may need additional lined paper (wider lines) and visual cues such as coloured dots in the margin and at the end of the line to know where to start and finish. This helps with spatial planning.

- Where excessive pressure is exerted, allow short breaks to relax the hand; also provide extra paper under their work to absorb pressure.

- Provide pens and pencils with integral rubber grips to ease strain. Consider chunky pens/pencils as less grip is required to hold these.

- Evaluate the use of a keyboarding scheme from the age of 9, which provides remedial and practical support.

- Place the paper to the side of the child's writing hand at an appropriate angle to ease the requirement to write across the body midline.

- Allow movement breaks for the child who finds sitting for extended periods mechanically uncomfortable. Consider use of a wobble cushion to allow movement/postural adjustment while seated.

- Provide templates where free drawing is not essential, and give positive feedback for effort made. Use of IT will be essential in secondary school if the child continues to have difficulties. Ensure that they have formal keyboard training prior to a senior school transition to allow use of a laptop to be integrated into lessons as and when appropriate.
- Limit frustration as much as possible by providing practical and positive verbal encouragement for the child.

Vision and eye movement control

What: definition and meaning

- It is estimated that approximately 70 to 80 per cent of our knowledge and perception of the world around us is obtained through our vision, and therefore good functioning of this system is vital in normal circumstances.

- Vision is the ability to take in sensory information through the eyes which is then sent to the brain's visual processing centres to be interpreted.

- The two eyes need to coordinate (work together) automatically and effortlessly with binocular vision in order to obtain a clear image to send to the brain's visual cortex, which processes the information.

- Some children with DCD/dyspraxia may have a reasonable optician's report (which evaluates acuity rather than the eyes working together), but when their eye movements are tested they may be unable to fix on and visually track a moving object in the horizontal or vertical plane, or easily move their eyes from one position to another. This has implications throughout their school day and for general life skills.

- Efficient motor control depends upon effective processing in the brain of the sensory inputs from the eyes, the balance system (both when static and when moving), sense of touch (tactile), body position (proprioceptive) awareness, and postural stability.

So what: issues and challenges

- Visual stress may result in the child rubbing or screwing up their eyes or covering up one eye to see adequately. They may experience headaches because of the eyestrain.

- The child may find it difficult to look at the board, particularly if sensitive to bright lighting, and their reaction to a white interactive board should be monitored.

- Fidgeting may occur as it is difficult for the child to maintain concentration and focus, with the eye discomfort causing distractibility when working.

◆ Tiredness and loss of concentration are common.

◆ There may be a general avoidance of close work by the child, or alternatively they may lean too close over their work, which can increase strain on the eye muscles.

◆ Abnormal postures may be observed when reading or writing.

◆ Blurring and/or doubling of print may be experienced by the child, particularly when tired at the end of the day.

◆ The child may experience difficulty in keeping their place and/or line when reading unless using their finger or a marker. Reading comprehension or accuracy may be compromised, and the child may develop a dislike of reading due to visual stress.

◆ Copying, either from book to paper or from board to paper, may be hard for them due to limited eye movement control in the vertical and horizontal planes, and due to difficulties moving their eyes from one position to another.

◆ Handwriting difficulties – poor spacing of letters in words and between words, erratic use of lines with letters incorrectly positioned; text may undulate and be difficult to read. Also, physical discomfort in the hand and forearm as well as fatigue may cause a reluctance to engage in written work.

◆ The child may exhibit poor coordination in ball games when catching, throwing, hitting with a bat, or kicking a ball due to reduced eye and hand coordination and/or an inability to visually track a moving ball or object.

◆ General frustration with school work and games due to reduced functioning may occur with a resultant loss of self-esteem for the child, particularly when they are innately intelligent.

Now what: practical strategies and ideas

Now what?

● Ensure that the child not only has an optician's report but also an examination by a behavioural optometrist to check their eye movements (functional vision). (See BABO in the 'Professional organisations' section.) Assessment and treatment should be under the remit of the National Health Service and at established opticians in the UK; similar resources can be sourced in other countries.

- An assessment by an occupational therapist offering a specific review of strengths and challenges is advisable. This should include checking dynamic and static balance, body awareness, and providing standardised tests of visual perception and visual motor integration to assist diagnosis.

- The above advice may also identify the possibility of a visual dyslexia.

- Ensure the child has good, shadow-free lighting and, where possible, natural lighting to work in. Monitor the effect of the interactive whiteboard on the child, particularly if they have sensory integrative issues (see Chapter 3). It is increasingly common for some children to have a heightened and sometimes adverse response to visual and auditory input.

- Ensure that the child sits facing the focus of teaching and/or the board to limit the amount of both eye and body movements when working between desk and board. Also, twisting or turning the body to locate from focus of teaching and back to the desk.

- The child should use an angled board to maximise forearm and wrist position as well as upright head position – this will help maintain good sitting posture, and aid visual movement between the board and desk, to reduce unnecessary fatigue. Alternatively, raise the desk up to at least elbow level to assist visual tracking between one plane and another.

- Provide short movement breaks to limit and ease visual strain when reading or writing for extended periods. Include changing the distance the eyes are focused on from near to far, as recommended for users of display screen equipment,.

- Allow some differentiation with printouts – using simple text such as Arial 12 point or ideally 14 point in bold print to minimise strain whenever possible.

- Extra time may be required for recording information – visual cues such as lined or graph paper may be required for writing.

- Allow the child to verbalise information in place of written work where appropriate in school lessons.

- Allow the child short breaks when working for extended periods at a computer or laptop. This will minimise any visual stress and consequent strain or overload on the child's sensory systems. Refer to the Display Screen Equipment (DSE)

Regulations produced by the Health and Safety Executive (www. hse.gov.uk). Establishing a visual break pattern in childhood will be beneficial for life as computer/screen use increases in work and home life.

- Make sure that the child achieves some personal success in ball games and PE by providing achievable goals; peer pair for extra practice in throwing, catching and bouncing a ball or hitting with a bat. For the younger child, a large balloon blown up to three-quarter size provides a valuable throwing and catching activity, as it allows time for them to plan and organise their eye and body movement response as the balloon moves more slowly than a ball. Balls with tails also help children visually track the path of a moving ball. Ensure the child knows that they need to watch the ball and follow its path to the hands or bat to enable success, this skill is often missed as it is assumed everyone instinctively knows to watch the ball. To increase the chances of success, use large targets to aim at, reducing them in size as success is achieved.

Handwriting

What: definition and meaning

Handwriting is a high level execution skill that brings together a whole range of complex sensory and motor abilities. Despite the increasing technology for recording information in children's lives, written work will still have a vital role to play. The following requirements underpin good handwriting but may present obstacles for those children who have not developed sound underlying sensory motor skills through play and other developmental opportunities. For example:

- Cognitive (mental) idea of what is required, motor planning and the ability to transfer information from the head to the page (execution).
- Adequate muscle tone and balance for postural stability and to maintain a consistent upright sitting position at a desk or work surface.
- The child's innate sense of their own body scheme and position in space and tactile (touch) feedback to inform them how hard they are gripping the pen and pressing on the paper.
- Functional eye movements to allow the child to scan and move their eye gaze from one position to another – for example, between the board and desk – and the ability to adjust their vision in both the horizontal and vertical planes.
- Integration of both sides of the body (bilateral integration) to allow the child to work and write across their body midline without having to twist, turn and adjust their body.
- Coordination and use of both hands together – one to write and the other to stabilise the work and make adjustments appropriately during writing.
- Integration/inhibition of the 'baby' or primitive reflexes which, if retained, can cause immature whole body and arm movement patterns in response to the child's head movements.
- Flexibility and isolation of movement between shoulder, arm, wrist and the muscles of the hands, fingers and thumb for fluidity of pen control and tool use.

- Smooth muscle control and mature 'dynamic' tripod grip with wrist slightly extended to facilitate cursive writing and to minimise any discomfort in the writing hand.
- Visual motor ability (looking and doing) affecting spatial orientation on paper, left/right, up/down and side to side.
- A good motor 'memory' of letter/number shape formation so cognitive monitoring is unnecessary and writing becomes automatic for the child.
- The 'just right' level of focus and attention for the task.
- Good listening and auditory processing skills.
- The ability to take in information from the environment, and filter and screen out unnecessary stimuli in order to give an appropriate response.
- Sequencing and organisational skills.

So what: issues and challenges

So what?

- The child may tire easily, tend to slump over their desk or head prop to maintain an upright position, and find extended writing an unpleasant experience. Frustration, task avoidance and stress may result.
- The child may not position themselves properly on the chair, tending to sit at an awkward angle, and not always know the pressure they are exerting through their hand when writing; their arm, hand and neck may ache.
- Poor feedback from the tactile (touch) and body awareness (proprioceptive) systems can also adversely affect the motor 'memory' of letters, numbers and shapes and automatic recall of how they are formed. The child then has to visually monitor their handwriting, usually at the expense of focusing on the content.
- Copying from the board or transferring information from one surface to another may be difficult, causing errors to be made and the child to fall behind in their work, despite their innate abilities.
- Hand preference may fluctuate if there is an unclear dominance. The child may also twist and turn in their seat or shift their body position as they find it difficult to work and write across their

body midline. (This may be caused by a lack of integration of both hemispheres of the brain and is not uncommon in some children with dyslexic tendencies.)

◆ Mechanical discomfort may be experienced when sitting in a flexed position at the desk, causing fidgeting. The child may feel the need to lean their head on their arms, extend their legs or sit on them to ease their 'mechanical' discomfort, but at the expense of their written work.

◆ Tremor and/or jerky movements may be observed. (Other conditions may manifest in this manner.) The child may struggle with coordinating their finger, thumb and hand movements and find manipulation and manual dexterity difficult and frustratingly slow.

◆ Whole arm movements may be observed in a range of everyday activities but particularly when writing, as the child is unable to isolate individual wrist, hand, finger and thumb movements. Recording information incurs much more effort for them than for their peers.

◆ Poor visual or motor spatial output on paper may be noted, and the child finds it difficult to position information correctly on the page. This difficulty is aggravated when the child has to turn round and then back again to their work in class. When drawing angles or changing direction on paper, for example, they may lose their orientation, resulting in the zigzagging of a shape (also a dyslexic tendency).

◆ The child may be easily distracted and lose focus as screening out background sounds is difficult for them.

◆ Verbal information may be hard to process or organise appropriately for writing information down, due to reduced auditory sequential memory (remembering things in order).

◆ The child may have a good ideation or thinking ability but not be able to organise, sequence and express ideas on paper in an automatic manner.

◆ Verbal skills may nevertheless be competent, and recording output can be considerably improved when a laptop or computer is introduced with the appropriate keyboard training. Keyboard training maximises the efficiency of typing by using all the digits. With practice, motor movements become automated through the development of 'muscle memory'. Typing where the user has to hunt for each letter is slow and time-consuming, requiring the focus to be on the typing at the expense of the content despite the child's knowledge and intelligence.

Now what: practical strategies and ideas

Now what?

- Allow some movement and stretching opportunities prior to sitting to alert the child's body position awareness. Encourage them to monitor and correct their own sitting position.
- The child's desk should be at or just below elbow height, with knees at 90 degrees with good lumbar support.
- The child should face the focus of teaching to minimise physical moving and shifting.
- Provision of an angled board as the writing surface might be necessary to allow correct positioning of the upper body, as when the head is bent over, the arms may also flex due to associated involuntary movement patterns, causing physical strain. A 20 degree angle is recommended for a laptop and for a writing slope for the correct ergonomic position to ease strain on the child's back and neck. (See Posturite and others in the 'Resources' section.)
- Release tension in forearms, hands and fingers and also increase awareness of arm position in space by encouraging the child to give their arms a gentle shake or clasp hands and stretch arms up into the air.
- Short built-in breaks should be provided to ease pressure on the writing hand. Provide integral textured pen grips to give feedback to grip.
- Check the child's functional vision with an optometrist to ensure that the muscle control of the eyes is functioning well, and that the writing on the board and their own written work are clear to them when adjusting their focus from one plane to another.
- Refine and improve fine motor coordination, finger isolation movement and control for handwriting. An assessment and an exercise programme should be sought from an appropriate therapist to mobilise and strengthen the hand and finger muscles.

- If possible, provide a therapy programme to build postural stability for trunk, shoulder and pelvic girdle under the direction of a physiotherapist or occupational therapist.

- Activities and games can be integrated into PE and free time to enhance spatial awareness, left and right orientation, symmetrical and cross-body pattern movements – all aspects of which are important for pen to paper activities.

- Visual cues, templates and stencils may be helpful in tandem with additional monitoring by a staff member to ensure success. Lined paper and enlarged graph paper may also assist in spatial challenges. Provide printed copies of notes to limit unnecessary written output.

- If handwriting becomes a severe challenge and does not reflect the child's innate ability, they may need to acquire and integrate keyboarding skills for schoolwork, particularly in secondary school, one or two years prior to the key examinations.

- A personal laptop may be required, and once the child has achieved a speed of approximately 20 to 25 words a minute, typewriting can be introduced to one or two key lessons with provision of a memory stick or appropriate technology for downloading information, including homework.

- The ability to type will allow the focus to be on expression of ideas rather than the child having to think about letter formation and pen control, assisting ideation. Paper and pen may still be required for effective planning of typed answers (e.g. mind maps/memory dumps), keeping this visible as the volume of typing increases.

- Typewriting is a remedial hand activity in its own right.

- Minimise extraneous sounds around the child and ensure some quiet time in class sessions. Avoid positioning near to thoroughfares but ensure they are facing the teacher/board/screen.

Additional tabletop handwriting exercises

The following exercises are designed to improve the range of hand movements and strength. They can be group or individual activities – 10 minute sessions, three times weekly.

1   The child (or children) should begin by shaking their hands and arms gently to relax them, ease any tension and alert the body awareness (proprioceptive) system.

2   Place forearms and hands palm down flat on the table with fingers placed together but extended (stretched out). Slowly spread fingers out into a fan shape then bring them back together. Do this at least three times.

3   With palms remaining face down on the table, curl fingers and thumb towards the palm of the hand into a tight fist, hold, then release to straighten – repeat three times.

4   Hands still on table, palms down, tap fingertips on the table:

   (a)   Make the sound of a horse walking.
   (b)   Make the sound of a horse trotting.
   (c)   Make the sound of a horse galloping.
   (d)   Relax hands by giving them another gentle shake and rest.

5   Using one hand at a time, place each finger in turn against the pad of the thumb, starting with the index (pointing) finger through to little finger and then back again. The child (or children) then try this with their eyes closed and/or with both hands working together.

6   Place forearms and hands back down onto the table. Keep elbows bent and practise turning hands over and back several times slowly. Ensure that the palms or the back of the hands are flat on the table before turning them back. Initially, this may incur associated arm and shoulder movements. Encourage the child to isolate the forearm and hand movements from the upper arm at the elbow. Practise this five or ten times. Once there is a movement rhythm, increase the speed, then slow down and stop.

7   Try activity 6, alternating the movement, with one palm face down and the other up, practising alternating movements with the object of creating smooth hand and forearm control.

Activities to improve pencil grasp

These exercises are designed for preschool and older children with coordination challenges, strengthening pincer grip between fingers and thumb.

Equipment and materials required:

- Short chunky chalks and chalkboard
- Chunky paintbrush
- Range of clothes pegs, shoe box or equivalent
- Real or pretend coins, money box or box with slot
- Beads or dried peas/beans, bottle with narrow neck
- Hollow pasta (which can be threaded and painted, shoelaces with extended tips (taped at the end if necessary to extend tip)
- Jacks or pebbles (washed)
- Old telephone directory or catalogue for tearing up
- Table tennis/ping pong balls
- Dried rice
- Chunky pegs and pegboards, posting games with counters
- Lego®, large size initially, reducing size as child becomes more competent.

1. **Use of chunky chalk for drawing on a board**

   - Use a vertical board to elevate the hand and forearm, and allow the fingers and thumb to fall into the correct pincer position around the chalk with the wrist slightly extended when the child is free drawing.
   - Helper to draw large shapes and letters on a chalkboard which the child can draw or paint over holding the barrel of a paintbrush in the preferred (dominant) hand. Reinforce the correct formation of letters and numbers, and encourage flowing lines, shapes and rhythm.

2. **Clipping pegs around a box**

- Buy different sized, shaped and coloured pegs.
- Clip the pegs around a shoe box or equivalent, and encourage the child to grip the pegs between finger and thumb using the least resistant pegs first.
- Practise squeezing and taking off the pegs using thumb and maybe two or three fingers initially, if the child cannot isolate finger and thumb movements.
- Progress to the child using their thumb and index finger – as their fingers get stronger, use each finger in turn against the pad of the thumb.
- The child can either do this on their own or take turns with a partner in a variety of games and activities, for example, 'peg dominoes'.
- Pegging items such as clothes to a suspended line, washing line style.

3. **Posting coins using a money box or container with a slot in it**

- Post the coins singly through the slot, ensuring the coins are picked up between the pads of the fingertips and thumb.
- It may be difficult for the child to orientate the position of the coin if they are under 4 years old due to less refined 'whole arm' movement control.

4. **Posting beads, dried beans or peas**

- Use a plastic bottle to avoid accidents and closely monitor the beads and peas for safety purposes for children aged 4 and under.

- The child should hold the bottle with their supporting hand and pick up peas/beans or beads one at a time to post through the top of the bottle.

- The child picks up the small objects between the thumb and index finger to post, then practises with each individual finger and the thumb, one at a time.
- Encourage use of both hands in each role as many activities in life demand some level of ability to work with both hands.
- Where there is a lack of clear hand preference in a younger child, position materials to the most preferred side to encourage more refined hand skills on one side, particularly for written output.

5. Pasta threading

- Use textured but hollow pasta. Keep in a dry container.
- Use a shoelace to thread the pasta together, ensuring that the individual pieces are picked up between the end pads of the finger and thumb.
- Encourage the child to use the same hand consistently by placing the pasta next to the hand the child writes with.

6. Jacks or pebbles (pebbles give a variety of textural feedback) – see therapeutic application below

These exercises are suitable for children aged 6 upwards.

- Practise bouncing a small ball and catching it without picking up the jacks/pebbles initially. Ensure that catching is successful over several attempts before attempting to pick up the jacks/pebbles and catch the ball at the same time.
- Pick up jacks one at a time after bouncing the ball and catching it at the same time. See how many jacks or pebbles the child can pick up in their hand by holding onto the ones in the palm while picking up others.

7. Old telephone directory or catalogue

- Tear out one or two sheets at a time with the 'writing' hand.
- Gather up and crush paper into a ball in one hand at a time.
- Use both hands together to make it into a tight ball.
- Throw the balls into a container or hoop with a consistent hand, again preferably the writing hand.

8. Rolling table tennis/ping pong balls

■ Use different coloured balls.

■ Line the balls up and place hand palm down; flick each one with the index finger over a marked line half a metre away (ideally on a smooth surface).

■ Repeat the activity with the other fingers doing the flicking.

9. Sticky/tacky rice

■ Place wet palm down on some dried rice in a container.

■ Turn hand over with the rice on top of the palm.

■ Use fingers and thumb to try to take the rice off the palm of the hand. (There may be some resistance from children with touch sensitivity.)

10. Pegs in pegboards

■ Use chunky pegs, picking them up between finger and thumb.

■ Make random patterns or copy from an original design. Talk about left/right, up/down, diagonal and side to side as the pegs are placed to incorporate spatial awareness.

11. Construction activity

■ Work with larger pieces of Lego® or a similar construction toy which offers little resistance and pressure. Progress to smaller pieces that also offer resistance as the child becomes more competent with manipulation.

■ Ensure that the child is successful in this activity by supporting where necessary, as they may have difficulty in visualising what they want to make or translating their ideas into action.

Jacks or fives: an example of a therapeutic application from a traditional game

Jacks or Fives requires:

- Understanding the sequence of the activity
- Motor planning and execution of the physical activity
- Eye and hand coordination
- Shoulder, forearm and wrist movement and control
- Grasp and release of hand and fingers at the correct moment
- Finger isolation movement when picking up the jacks
- Timing of the sequence of the task
- Using the right force to bounce the ball appropriately
- Fluency of movement
- An automatic motor adaptive response to the bouncing of the ball.

The activity should be broken down into small achievable steps as with any new activity, and time should be given for each part. For example, allow the child to practise bouncing and catching the ball for several minutes until achieved before attempting to pick up the jacks, one at a time initially, progressing to two, three, four and five at a time.

Scissor skills

What: prerequisites

What?

■ Well-maintained safety scissors or adapted scissors (see PETA UK and Taskmaster in the 'Resources' section). Left-handed scissors may be required.

The child requires:

■ Reasonable shoulder and trunk stability.
■ The ability to coordinate both hands together for use: bilateral integration.
■ A consistent dominant hand to place the scissors in and a stabilising or supporting hand to hold the paper or card.
■ The opportunity to sit at an elbow height table to steady elbows for cutting.
■ The ability to isolate finger and thumb movements in order to hold the scissors with the thumb in the upper hole grip and the fingers below prior to cutting.
■ Sufficient hand and finger strength and dexterity to manipulate and cut out the shape.
■ Reasonable body position feedback from arms and hands.
■ Adequate visual perceptual and visual motor skills to identify and then cut round a shape appropriately.

So what: issues and challenges

So what?

◆ Trunk and shoulder stability may be weak, making it difficult for the child to steady their arms and control the scissors.
◆ The child may not be able to hold standard scissors due to reduced motor control and limited finger and thumb movements.
◆ The child may not have the ability to coordinate and use both hands together or have a clear hand preference for cutting.

◆ The child may elevate elbows out to the side (as with the use of a knife and fork), attempting to cut 'in the air' as a result of difficulty in isolating forearm and hand movements, thus limiting control of the scissors and card. (This is sometimes seen in children with a retained asymmetrical tonic neck reflex.)

◆ If the child has reduced or low muscle tone, they may find it difficult to exert sufficient pressure on the scissors or to isolate finger movements.

◆ A reduced sense of arm and hand position in space will make cutting unpredictable and poorly controlled, and pressure may vary on the scissors.

◆ The child may have difficulty with integrating the visual and motor aspects of the tasks and have a poor spatial awareness.

◆ A combination of the above challenges may incur frustration and result in avoidance of cutting and allied tasks.

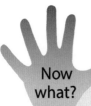

Now what?

Now what: practical strategies and ideas

■ Assess for and provide a choice of safety and/or adapted scissors to evaluate the child's best performance – for example, the Taskmaster scissor assessment kit (see the 'Resources' section).

■ Allow the child to undertake a simple stretching exercise with hands clasped and arms above the head to 'wake up' their body awareness. Alternatively, ask the child to gently shake and relax their arms and hands.

■ The helper should evaluate and break down the activity into small achievable steps.

■ The table should be at the child's elbow height with work placed symmetrically in front of the child and their elbows placed on the table to stabilise their work and provide postural stability.

■ Ensure that the child is helped to position fingers and thumbs correctly prior to cutting, with the thumb placed through the top hole of the scissors and the elbows stabilised to stop the child lifting them up.

- The child can practise cutting by snipping up plastic straws to achieve the correct cutting action. A collage can be made of different coloured straws for the young child.

- Allow the child to practise with thick card and wider lines initially to ensure success. Start with straight lines, then simple angles and curves, and finally complex shapes to ensure success.

- Allow short breaks and gentle stretching of the hands and fingers if the activity is extended and the child tires.

- Give positive feedback and encouragement for the effort made, even if it is not to the required standard (yet!).

- The advice of an occupational therapist may be required in tandem with the evaluation of other fine motor, visual perceptual and visual motor skills if the child has been struggling with a range of manual tasks, particularly handwriting.

- Exercises for postural strengthening and stability, eye and hand coordination and to promote integration of both sides of the body may be necessary, with a referral made to a physiotherapist or occupational therapist if there are ongoing concerns for the child's upper limb motor skills.

- Checking of the child's eyesight may be necessary by a local optician, who can be asked to assess functional vision if the child continues to have difficulty with practical desktop tasks. Consider assessment by a behavioural optometrist, as previously noted, as challenges with higher level skills can indicate other un-recognised difficulties.

Chapter 5

Visual perception

Visual perceptual difficulties

What: definition and meaning

What?

(See also the sections on visual motor integration and vision and eye movement control in the previous chapter.)

Visual perception is the ability to take in information from the environment via our eyes. The information is integrated, processed and interpreted by the brain to allow the child to give an appropriate response, as, for example, in reading and writing. If visual processing is weak or fragmented, it is much harder for a child to make sense of the incoming visual information and respond appropriately.

The various aspects of visual perception cannot easily be separated from each other, but for purposes of understanding specific issues a child may experience, they are normally subdivided into the following:

■ Visual discrimination: the ability to look at and match a shape with an identical one picked out from a group of other similar shapes.
■ Visual spatial perception: the ability to recognise a single shape in a group of identical shapes that has a part or the whole of it going in a different direction.
■ Visual memory (also has a cognitive component): the ability to hold the memory of a shape for several seconds and then match it with the identical shape within a group of similar shapes.
■ Visual sequential memory (also has a cognitive component): the ability to remember progressively longer sequences of shapes for a few seconds and match them with the correct group out of several options.

- Visual figure ground perception: the ability to recognise a shape and then find the same shape hidden in the background of a range of lines and patterns.
- Visual closure: the ability to look at a shape and match it with one of several incomplete shapes which would be identical if completed.
- Visual form constancy: the ability to look at a shape and then find it in a group of other shapes, although it may be larger, smaller, turned around or reversed.

Visual discrimination

Visual discrimination is the ability to look at and match a shape with an identical one picked out from a group of other shapes. Here the shapes and forms remain constant, so it is primarily the recognition and matching of identical shapes.

So what: issues and challenges

So what?

◆ A child with difficulty in visual discrimination is likely to struggle across the range of visual perceptual tasks and with most aspects of schoolwork – for example, recognising and interpreting simple or more complex shapes such as the difference between the letters 'K' and 'R' or the words 'was' and 'saw'.

◆ The child may have difficulties in both interpreting visual information and/or reproducing it accurately, such as when copying from a smartboard in school.

◆ The child may need additional support and cues with these tasks despite their innate intelligence.

Now what: practical strategies and ideas

Now what?

● Ensure that a full optician's evaluation is undertaken between the ages of 5 and 7. Also seek the advice of an optometrist who can check functional eye movement skills – see the previous chapter for symptoms of visual 'stress'.

● An occupational therapy assessment which includes a full visual perceptual evaluation may be required to identify the key areas of challenge for the child. The occupational therapist can advise whether the challenges are primarily with visual perception or with motor output – the latter is usually more common in children with dyspraxia. It may, however, be a combination of both.

● Use a 'multi-sensory' approach of look, see, say, along with handling of shapes and objects, to allow the brain to process information through different senses. If one area is weak another may compensate, using a different pathway in the brain to access learning.

- Allow the child to think and speak about the different qualities of a variety of objects in relation to texture, size and shape. Help them to make up different matching shapes, using games such as Guess Who, Tap a Shape and Lego® designs that can be printed off from its website.
- Draw a shape with a finger on the child's hand (hidden) or back and ask them to identify it; they then repeat the activity with their partner.
- Play a variety of card games such as Snap with different topic cards, matching 'pairs'. Dobble is a great game for visual discrimination; make use of the resources available in toyshops to address this specific area.

Visual spatial perception

Visual spatial perception is the ability to recognise and match an existing shape with another in a group of similar shapes that has part or all of it going in a different direction from the rest.

So what: issues and challenges

- The child with visual spatial dysfunction may appear poorly coordinated, disorganised and tend to bump into things due to a reduced sense of where their own body is in relation to the environment and others around them.
- The child may find ball games difficult as they have problems judging the distance and speed of the ball travelling through space. They also have difficulty aiming at a target or with any activity which needs a sense of distance, as when hitting a ball in tennis or playing netball.
- Fine motor skills may be difficult for the child – for example, doing up shoelaces and playing with Lego®. They may also have difficulty with concepts of left and right and demonstrate poor directional sense both in motor activities and on paper.
- Letter formation may be messy due to directional confusion and inconsistent letter size and spacing.
- The child may have difficulty in working from left to right on paper in a consistent manner and lose their orientation, or the writing drifts across the page. Other problems may include copying from the board, letter or number recognition and reversals, as in children with dyslexic tendencies.
- The child may have difficulty working out the underlying spatial orientation of written and drawn work – for example, maths layout, position of numbers and again the orientation on paper.

Now what: practical strategies and ideas

- The child should face the board and focus of teaching in class as they may find it hard to transfer information across the two planes from board (vertical) to paper (horizontal) – see also vision and eye movement control in Chapter 4.

- The child's desktop should be as clear as possible with only the materials required for the immediate task to hand. Use of a 'see-through' pencil case will assist planning and organisation.

- The child can be helped by copying from information next to them on the desk where appropriate (use Arial 12 to 14 point for clarity). An individual whiteboard or tablet and stylus can be useful tools.

- The child may need extra time for planning and organisation to enable them to remain calm and minimise stress.

- Provide the child with colour-coded folders for different subjects, which can be cross-referenced on the visual (laminated) timetable.

- Use 'squared' paper (enlarged for the younger child) for pen and pencil work where possible to provide cues for the orientation of work on paper.

- Provide the child with a multi-sensory approach to spatial concepts using items such as pencils and rulers and games to demonstrate 'in, on, next to, in front of'.

- Use markers from left to right to indicate where the (younger) child should begin and end written work – green for start and red for stop – until it becomes automatic for them. Allow extra time for recording.

- For younger children 'dot to dot', tracing, stencils and other fun activities can help directionality and position on paper and facilitate manual dexterity and resultant pen skills.

- Pattern copying using magnets, pegs, Connect Four, Lego® and similar activities are useful. Assist the child as required to follow instructions on construction activities and to learn to carry written information from instructions across to the activity (ideation, motor planning and execution).

- Homework could include an activity to enhance spatial and mathematical skills using construction games as a medium. This provides a multi-sensory approach to learning when the child is supported to take an interest and learn new 'adaptive' responses.

- It is easy to adapt ball games for a child with visual spatial difficulties. Here are some examples: practise catching and throwing chiffon scarfs, balloons or balls with bells inside; targeting a ball at a wall and catching it on its return; throwing and catching beanbags, or large and small balls at different speeds.

Visual memory and visual sequential memory

Visual memory is the ability to hold the memory of a shape for several seconds and then match it with the same shape within a group of similar shapes. Visual sequential memory is the ability to remember progressively longer sequences of shapes for a few seconds and match them with the same group out of several options. Thus, there is a cognitive component to these two aspects of visual perception.

So what: issues and challenges

So what?

◆ The child may have difficulties with reading, as well as remembering visual sequences of letter or number shapes.

◆ Taking notes and copying from a board may be difficult for the child as they cannot retain the information in working memory.

◆ The child may not be able to remember and carry over information from one visual activity to another, or reproduce symbols and information, which can become a source of frustration and stress.

◆ The child may have difficulty sequencing letters and numbers correctly on the page.

◆ The child may find concentration and focus on a task difficult to sustain.

◆ Planning and organising work may be difficult for the child, as well as remembering work and information learned previously.

◆ Visual memory recall may fluctuate from day to day as with other aspects of dyspraxia, and may lack consistency in general application both at home and in school.

◆ The older child may find they have to keep checking visual information – for example, signs and directions – as visual recall is inconsistent.

◆ The child may experience anxiety, run out of time and miss appointments due to organisational and sequencing deficits.

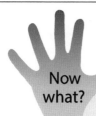

Now what?

Now what: practical strategies and ideas

- Ensure that the child faces the teacher in order to both hear and observe what they are saying – this allows a multi-sensory method for retaining information and reinforcement for remembering information.
- Reinforce information, especially for homework, in written form – check that the child has written down the correct instructions in their home/school book.
- Allow extra time for copying from the board and general recording, as a child with visual memory challenges may have to check information several times, as well as having to deal with the 'mechanics' of handwriting.
- Provide the younger child with graph paper of different sizes to assist in numbers, letters and shapes being placed in the correct orientation.
- Encourage the whole class to be quieter when engaged in copying work from the board to limit distraction.
- Provide an outline sequential format for planning written projects and a large (12 to 14 point) Arial timetable; keep with their core workbooks and up to date. Work through it with the child at home.

Activities for primary school:
- Use fun perceptual motor activities which encourage the child to remember a sequence of directions – for example, copying or tracing colours and shapes. This may help them to hold visual information in working memory.
- Provide a tray of four to six familiar items. The child looks at them for five to ten seconds; then cover the tray after removing one item at a time and ask the child to recall what is missing from the tray.
- Arrange four or five objects in order, then mix them up and ask the child to place them back in order.
- Draw three or four different shapes, letters or numbers on the board and then erase. Ask the child to draw or say what they saw.
- Muddle comic strip or other sequential activities and ask the child to place them back in order.
- Pegboard games: make up patterns for the child to copy or create a design from existing templates in a game.

Visual figure ground perception

Visual figure ground perception is the ability to draw out important visual information from other background information.

So what: issues and challenges

So what?

◆ The child may find it difficult to screen out unnecessary background stimuli, thus losing focus on the main task, object or symbol.

◆ The child may become easily distracted and taken off task.

◆ When reading the child may lose their place, due to scanning difficulties and visual confusion, especially when copying from the board.

◆ The child may struggle to find a place on a map, or in written work, due to all the other background information drawing their attention.

◆ The organisation of the child's work may be poor on paper.

◆ Depth perception may be poor and the child may be accident-prone as they misjudge the distance of objects in relation to their background – for example, when reaching for a cup or object. When playing games or in PE, the child may struggle to identify key objects such as a ball from the general background.

Now what: practical strategies and ideas

Now what?

● See information in the section on visual discrimination above and vision and eye movement control (Chapter 4) for advice with regard to the child's functional vision.

● Minimise clutter around the child's workstation and on the board.

● Simplify presentation of work to be copied and allow additional time for this activity.

● Provide verbal prompts and cues and additional help if the child is struggling.

- Assist with scissor work if the child has difficulty maintaining line position. Provide thicker paper and/or wider, coloured lines for clearer definition to practise cutting.
- Clearly label materials and keep them in a consistent place for ease of access by the child.
- Games such as Dig In, Pick Up Sticks and sorting activities such as different coloured buttons, sorting different shapes of dried pasta, and circling specific letters on a worksheet can help to strengthen this skill.

Visual closure

Visual closure is the ability to look at a shape, then work out which one of several incomplete shapes would be the same, if fully completed.

So what: issues and challenges

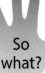

So what?

◆ When reading, a child may normally only perceive the partial shape of the letter and the brain then 'fills in' the rest of the letter (conceptualising), thus allowing the child to read more fluently. This is difficult for the child with a poor underlying concept of letter and number shapes, and they need constant multi-sensory reinforcement.

◆ The child with poor visual closure may find spelling difficult, as it requires the matching up of several component parts to make a whole word.

◆ When part of a shape is missing or occluded, the child may not be able to recognise the whole shape as their brain is unable to recall a whole shape pattern without all the information.

◆ Visualising images as a whole may be difficult for the child, and they may not 'recall things' to mind – for example, when trying to picture how get to from one place to another (geographical orientation). Map reading may also be difficult for the older child.

◆ The child may not be able to match individual parts together from a whole constructional activity – for example, a jigsaw – in order to make up the complete pattern. They cannot visualise the whole or see an overview.

◆ Calculations for maths and multiplication tables may be difficult.

◆ Gaining the sense of the 'whole picture' for planning and organisation purposes may be a challenge in the flow of the day at school or at home.

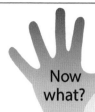

Now what: practical strategies and ideas

- Enlarge the written word when the child is learning to read fluently – stories should be short enough to hold interest. Allow the child to break down new words into the sounds of the letters and reinforce this at the end of the session. Give positive feedback for effort made as opposed to purely the end results.

- Provide extra support for spelling and recognition of new and more complex words.

- Allow the child to handle and manipulate shapes to give touch feedback when asked to explain the properties of objects.

- Provide jigsaw puzzles at the level where a child is successful, which may not always match their chronological age, allowing time when there is a peer or adult around to direct the child's focus and interest.

- Cut up simple pictures, ideally of a subject that the child has a particular interest in. The child can then arrange them and glue them back together.

- Present a selection of enlarged incomplete patterns or shapes which the child can trace with their finger and describe what is missing.

- The teacher partially covers a picture and asks the child to describe the whole picture in their own words. Also draw half a picture on a folded piece of paper and then ask the child to draw the other half.

- 'Dot to dot' using pictures with either numbers or letters – the teacher asks the child to guess what the picture will be at some point before completion.

- Help the child to construct three-dimensional models from Lego® or similar construction toys, encouraging them to describe what they are planning.

- Ask the child to fill in squares, triangles, diamonds and other more complex and incomplete shapes.

- The teacher provides stencil patterns (including letter and number patterns) for the child to fill in freehand. These can be the plastic stencils, which give clear boundaries, card cut-out stencils or worksheets with patterns on.

- See the 'Resources' section for Ann Arbor Publishers and Happy Puzzle Company.

Visual form constancy

Visual form constancy is the ability to look at a shape and then recognise it in a group of other shapes, although it may be larger, smaller, turned around or reversed.

So what: issues and challenges

So what?

◆ The child may struggle to interpret written information on a board – copying may be difficult, especially when rapid changes of information are made.

◆ The teachers' varying styles of handwriting may present problems due to different sizing and change in basic letter formation, particularly with cursive writing.

◆ The child may find sorting and understanding the properties of objects, shapes and symbols difficult.

◆ Altering of shapes and forms or putting them in different positions may be difficult for the child and cause them confusion, particularly when asked to draw them or describe their properties.

◆ The child may find construction activities hard – for example, using two-dimensional information and then translating it into a three-dimensional construction activity.

Now what: practical strategies and ideas

Now what?

● The teacher should help to minimise clutter around the child's working area and on the board.

● The teacher should ensure consistency with written work for the child to copy; when printing information out, where possible use a consistent typeface (such as Arial 12 or 14 point).

● Alert other teaching staff to the fact that the child is likely to recognise the printed word more easily than different styles of cursive writing.

● Give additional support to the child in design and technology activities.

- Use the many resources in children's books to match and link shapes that are larger or smaller or in a different position.
- Think of a shape – for example, a square, circle or triangle – and ask the child to find similar shapes in the room around them. Match visual shapes with actual shapes that the child explores with their hands.
- The teacher turns shapes around and puts them in different positions and sees if the child can recognise them – overlap them with other shapes for increased difficulty.
- The child is asked to identify which is the larger, smaller, thicker, thinner, etc. between a pair of objects. Start at the level at which they are successful and then make the differences more subtle.
- The teacher writes the same word in many styles, colours and prints, together with a range of other words. The child identifies and underlines the one word.
- The teacher encourages the child to match two-dimensional shapes on paper with three-dimensional objects using different perceptual shapes and puzzles appropriate to their functional level.
- The teacher provides a clearly printed sheet of writing and asks the child to pick out lower and upper case letters.
- Provide computer activities which focus on discrimination of different shapes and symbols. Ask the child to trace over squares, circles and triangles, and then copy them onto a chalkboard (for the younger child).
- The child strings or lays out beads or buttons of one shape that vary in size or colour. The child also copies shapes on a pegboard from varying design layouts.
- Provide the child with the 'just right' level of support and motivation to engage in all the activities for visual perception and make it fun, especially for the younger child!

Additional visual perceptual activities for the younger child

■ Allow the child to trace simple shapes from a book and cut them out.

■ Provide sorting games using objects of different sizes, colour, shape and texture.

■ Encourage 'I Spy' games for younger children on walks and around the house, picking out particular objects or shapes from the background.

■ Help the child to pick out different leaf shapes on a nature walk, or recognise different grasses and sedges (use 'I Spy' books).

■ Books such as *Where's Wally* are fun ways to isolate a shape from the background.

■ Provide games such as bead threading, making collages and jigsaw puzzles, but with a shared involvement and at the right 'functional' level to maintain the child's interest.

Jigsaw puzzle – a simple activity to enhance visual perception, requiring:

■ Visual discrimination – recognising the relevant parts.

■ Form constancy – seeing and recognising the shapes in different positions.

■ Figure ground perception – drawing out the relevant visual information from a background of information.

■ Spatial ability – recognising the orientation of one shape to another.

■ Visual closure – recognising the whole shape when still incomplete.

■ Sequential memory – holding information in working memory when looking around for the relevant piece(s).

■ Fine motor manipulation and manual dexterity including good pincer grip between the finger and thumb.

■ Light touch control.

- Patience and ability to stay on task.
- Concentration and attention.

Ensure that the jigsaw puzzle is at the 'just right' challenge level for the individual child and that someone is with them to encourage their interest.

Chapter 6

Bilateral integration sequencing (BIS)

Organising and working both sides of the body together

This picture was automatically drawn by a child with average intelligence during an assessment, and appears to reflect an innate but unconscious lack of integration between the two sides of their body.

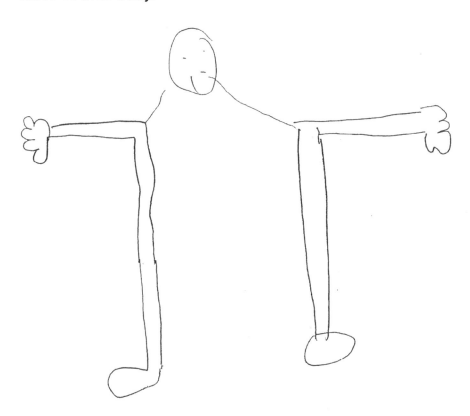

Bilateral integration: an overview

What?

What: definition and meaning

Bilateral integration is the ability to coordinate and work both sides of the body together at the same time for use in everyday activities. It develops within the first five to seven years of life, and requires an area of the brain known as the corpus callosum to mature completely, The corpus collosum connects the two sides or hemispheres of the brain *and* has the job of facilitating or inhibiting all the information passed between them . Where the connections between both sides of the brain are poor, one side of the body can appear to work almost independently from the other. This makes it difficult for a child to integrate the two sides of the body together for many day-to-day activities.

So what?

So what: issues and challenges

◆ The child may not have a consistent right- or left-sided hand, foot, ear or eye preference when picking up a pen, kicking a ball, using a phone or looking through a telescope or camera lens.

◆ The child may start to write or draw across the paper to their body midline, but then pass the pencil to the other hand to finish their work across the page (this is often noted in preschool children before integration is complete).

◆ Some children cannot physically write or work across their body midline. As a result, the child may twist or rotate their body or shift to one side on their chair (see additional information on the asymmetrical tonic neck reflex in Chapter 7).

◆ In tests of manual dexterity, the child may have hands that are equally able to perform fine motor tasks as opposed to one more dextrous hand, but cannot fully refine one side for manual tasks such as handwriting.

◆ When writing, the child may 'forget' that they have two hands and neglect the supporting or stabilising arm, leaving it down by their side.

- The child may find it difficult to orientate one hand to another and be unsure which hand should 'lead' when, for example, tying a knot, using a knife and fork, or doing up shoelaces and buttons.
- Reduced coordination may be observed for reciprocal (cross-pattern) movements such as climbing and skipping and riding a bicycle. The child may run in an ungainly manner, and also have difficulty in coordinating their upper body with the lower body – particularly in swimming and allied sports.
- An involuntary 'blink' may be observed at the midline of the body when the child is visually tracking a moving object with their eyes in the horizontal plane.
- Where there is no clear eye dominance, reading and general processing of visual information may be difficult. When the child tries to look through a telescope, for example, they may be unsure which eye to use. (This can also be due to a reduced sense of their body scheme – see the section on proprioception in Chapter 3.)

Now what: practical strategies and ideas

Now what?

- In class the teacher or assistant can prompt the child to place their helping hand on the work surface within their visual field to stabilise the paper when working. Prompts can be verbal or visual, but regular reminders are important to encourage the child to involve both hands for everyday tasks.
- Encourage a consistent writing and leading hand by placing materials on the dominant side. Remind the child to stabilise their work with the non-dominant hand.
- If the child has a clear one-sided dominance (laterality) but finds it difficult to work across the body midline, their work can also be placed on the dominant side to avoid any compensatory twisting and turning.
- An occupational therapist can provide an overall assessment to assist in identifying which would be the preferred hand if this remains unclear in the primary school child. Advice can also be provided on appropriate therapy.

- Encourage the child to use both sides of their body together in a range of symmetrical activities such as jumping with both feet together, hand-clapping activities, skipping exercises, holding onto a baton with both hands to hit a balloon backwards and forwards, as a precursor to working with reciprocal cross-pattern movements. Games and activities such as lacing, threading and using building blocks are fun and encourage the hands to work together, crossing midline can also be encouraged.

- Opportunities for extra time to practise functional skills such as the use of a knife and fork and managing buttons and tying shoelaces should be integrated into the child's day so that they are not put under pressure at key times.

- Bilateral integration challenges are likely to affect the child's functional eye skills. While many children may have had a successful optician's test, the functional movements of their eyes may not have been tested. The advice of an optometrist should be sought as this can make a considerable difference to the child's function in school. See BABO in the 'Professional organisations' section at the end of this book.

Organisational and sequencing skills

What: definition and meaning

What?

This area commonly presents a considerable challenge to some children with dyspraxia. The abilities to organise and sequence activities are interdependent and require the child to have clear ideation, planning and executive (output) abilities for everyday tasks.

Sensory motor integration as a foundation to organisation and sequencing abilities involves the following:

- In a child's early years there is considerable expansion of all the neural circuitry and connections in the brain.
- As the child grows, many of these connections are refined or 'pruned', allowing the remaining connections to mature and become 'hard wired' or more fully laid down.
- The child's sensory systems of vision, hearing, smell, taste, sense of touch, body awareness and balance need to become fully integrated in order for the child to function and access higher level skills such as organisation and sequencing.

So what: issues and challenges

So what?

- In some children there will be an underlying impairment of both sensory and motor organisation, making it difficult for them to respond appropriately to the demands placed on them both at home and at school.
- The child may not be able to think and therefore plan in a logical sequence, affecting their ability to get their inherently good ideas down on paper. They may have a good ideation of what they want to say or write, but planning and/or execution of the activity is compromised.
- The child's work may be messy and untidy with poor spatial presentation, as they have to battle with reduced manual dexterity and manipulation for writing and drawing, as well as coping with their organisational challenges.

◆ It may be hard for the child to prioritise thoughts, and they are easily taken off task and distracted from the activity in hand. Holding information in working memory in an orderly sequence may be a component of this: the child may appear forgetful and generally disorganised.

◆ The child may struggle to plan ahead in everyday activities and have difficulty organising themselves and their belongings.

◆ If the child is given two or three instructions, the first may be successful but the others 'forgotten', and the child can easily become sidetracked onto another activity.

◆ Auditory sequential memory and/or visual sequential memory may be difficult for the child, as well as working through a sequence of tasks. Holding short-term information in working memory may also be weak as a result.

◆ The child may also miss the relevant point in what is being asked of them unless the question or request is directed specifically to them and then repeated.

◆ Timing may be poor in responding to requests, and the child may appear inattentive and distracted.

◆ The child is likely to leave equipment and materials behind, or take longer to organise their school belongings, when others are ready to attend to the next step.

◆ There may be a degree of generalised anxiety and frustration as it is hard for the child and others around them to understand why everyday tasks take so long and why the child always seems to be one step behind others.

Now what?

Now what: practical strategies and ideas

● Ideally, therapeutic advice and activities should be provided for children at primary school age, in tandem with advice from an occupational therapist experienced in sensory integration in order to address any underlying sensory and motor developmental immaturities.

● There is likely to be a 'mismatch' between the child's innate intelligence and their reduced performance. Provide positive feedback for effort shown in school and home activities as self-esteem may be low, causing frustration and anger. The child needs to be supported positively to minimise the impact poor organisational and sequencing skills can cause.

- The child's attention should be fully gained when being given instructions. Also avoid giving too many instructions at one time as this can cause confusion.

- Specific activities that the child finds difficult may need some actual 'hands on' help: for example, organising paperwork and planning the flow of the day. See the 'Resources' section – IANSYST Ltd has valuable tools for children with organisational and sequencing issues.

- Multi-sensory reinforcement of instructions both verbally and visually – for example, print outs, information written up on board and the use of a keyboard – can be valuable. Ensure adequate information is taken down by the child to allow success in homework and other projects.

- Mind maps, extra planning time and a prepared format giving cues for what the child needs to consider when planning a project can assist.

- Ensure that the child has well-maintained writing and recording tools and strategies such as a 'see-through' pencil case to allow quick checking of equipment. Also work topics should be colour-coded and/or kept together in individual folders. The colour-coding can be cross-referenced on a written timetable.

- The acquisition of keyboard skills prior to secondary school can provide an excellent strategy to enable a child with a recognised dyspraxia to organise their thoughts and ideas on paper as this enables efficient editing. Providing the child has gained competent keyboard skills of 20 to 25 words a minute, the use of a laptop can be gradually integrated into appropriate lessons with a view to using this strategy for higher level examinations.

- A watch with a clear face is vital: in secondary school a mobile phone or PDA (personal digital assistant) is valuable for reminders or main appointments. The child may need additional time for organising each transition in class.

- At home ensure that school clothes are laid out ready the night before and contents of the school bag checked against a visual timetable, the latter placed where the child can easily refer to it. Ensure updates are maintained for any changes.

Additional games and activities to facilitate organisation, sequencing and working memory

These can be integrated as part of a PE lesson or games.

- Obstacle races which can be adapted to provide as much variety as possible, involving left and right, through, round, up and over, to facilitate spatial organisation.
- Ball bouncing, catching, throwing games in pairs or groups taking turns – focusing on left and right, up and down, side to side and counting.
- Charades, mime and dance sequences.
- Hopscotch can be adapted for a variety of sequential activities, including hopping and jumping backwards, forwards and side to side.
- Card games such as Pairs, Snap, Rummy, Knock-out Whist and Solitaire.
- Traditional games including Noughts and Crosses, Snakes and Ladders, dominoes, chess, strategic peg games, Kim's Game for working memory (see the Happy Puzzle Company in the 'Resources' section).
- Construction games and building games.
- Cartoon books/magazines for visual sequencing.
- Typing skills to a level of 30 words a minute for secondary school.
- Piano or other musical instruments.
- Horse riding, particularly involving indoor schooling.
- Indoor 'Clip' n' Climb' or outdoor climbing and/or bouldering.
- Activities under the direction of an occupational therapist for sensory motor integration.

Concentration and attention

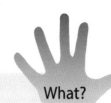

What: definition and meaning

■ The ability to maintain focus, concentration and attention, and to sit still and quietly is the result of a 'symphony' of integration within a child's sensory motor system. Children with dyspraxia may lack integration due to underlying developmental immaturity, which will affect their ability to concentrate and attend to the task in hand.

■ The frontal area of the brain which supports cognition, impulse control, decision-making, focus and attention may not have fully matured and integrated, making it particularly challenging for children whose schooling begins at a very early age.

■ The maturity of the vestibular (balance) system is key to enabling the child is at the right level of 'arousal' and focus, with both sides of the brain working together for optimum learning.

■ Sensory processing challenges may cause the child to lack concentration and attention due to difficulty in filtering out all the sensory information they receive through their tactile (touch), visual (looking) and auditory (listening) systems. These systems may be hypersensitive, affecting the child's ability to concentrate because of all the additional stimulation they are having to deal with.

So what: issues and challenges

◆ Children with dyspraxia or an underlying developmental coordination disorder can lack the cortical or brain inhibition for impulse and attention control and be easily taken off task. The child may be a 'dreamer' or easily distracted by their own thoughts.

◆ The child's underlying organisational and sequencing skills may be poor and their level of output and written work may be adversely affected.

◆ Children with sensory integrative dysfunction may also experience a reduced awareness of their own body position in space, affecting their level of concentration and focus.

- ◆ The child's touch system may be over- or under-reactive, causing sensitivity to clothes textures and physical contact with other children, for example. This in turn can adversely affect their concentration on the task in hand in class.

- ◆ If the child has a heightened awareness of what is going on around them in terms of visual and sound distraction, especially in a busy classroom, the lack of concentration and attention can be exacerbated when the child is placed facing their peers as opposed to the focus of teaching.

- ◆ Vision and hearing may be heightened and acutely sensitive, causing distractibility (see the Moro reflex in the Chapter 7). The child may be alert to sounds that are normally filtered out by others and not be able to distinguish the relevant incoming stimuli from the teacher or environment around them, causing them considerable distraction.

- ◆ It is important to ensure that the child has sufficient water throughout the day as dehydration can lead to lack of concentration. Ensure that the child has slow release high-fibre foods, particularly at the beginning and middle of the day to maintain energy levels. Nutritional advice can also be sought, as some children who are low on essential nutrients such as omega 3s and iron, for example, can display poor concentration and attention.

- ◆ For those children with the more severe attention deficit (and hyperactivity) disorders – a condition sometimes seen overlapping with dyspraxia – medication is occasionally prescribed. The long-term effects of this are not yet clearly known, and support and advice on aspects of sensory processing can assist as an alternative technique.

Now what?

Now what: practical strategies and ideas

- ● Whole class teaching is valuable where there can be shared quiet periods during the lesson to minimise distraction.

- ● The child's desk should face the teacher and the board to avoid turning between board and desk and the attendant distractions, particularly if the child's short-term auditory and/or visual retention is poor.

- Give time for planning and organisation of materials at the beginning of each task to avoid increasing the child's stress levels, as this can help them to settle and concentrate.
- Break down verbal and written instructions into simple steps, with a clear beginning, middle and end. Give reminders of what is to happen next. Minimise visual clutter on the desk and board where possible.
- Allow a multi-sensory approach to enable the child to use their best personal learning methods – for example, visual, auditory, tactile or kinaesthetic, or a combination for the younger child. If one channel for learning is weak, then others can be used in a compensatory manner to support learning skills.
- Minimise noise levels and movement around the child. Avoid placing a child with limited focus and attention span next to a window or in the main thoroughfare.
- Where possible, provide times of quiet where there can be complete attention on task to build up the ability to work for longer periods.
- Colour-code different subject books, use a 'see-through' pencil case so that materials can be seen at a glance and maintain the child's ability to feel in control.
- A child may be unable to transfer information across two planes: that is, between board (vertical) and paper (horizontal) – especially if eye movements are poor. It is helpful to put notes on the desk and/or allow extra time for recording information to limit stress and anxiety.
- Minimise pressure on the child and anxiety by giving positive feedback for the effort made during the lesson.
- Allow movement opportunities for children who are fidgety – for example, to give papers out – to ease any postural discomfort, which is common in children with an underlying coordination disorder.
- Allow a child with 'touch' sensitivity sufficient space to avoid unnecessary nudging and bumping as the child may overreact to physical contact.
- More unusually, if a child has occasional 'absences' and seems 'disconnected' from what is going on around them, resulting in a complete lack of response, this can sometimes indicate underlying mild seizure activity and should be monitored closely with a view to referring for a medical opinion. This is obviously different from being 'off task' or experiencing a general loss of attention or concentration.

Chapter 7

Primitive or baby reflexes

Overview

What: definition and meaning

What?

- Reflexes are early inbuilt automatic movement patterns, some of which start in the womb, and are a normal part of early development.

- These primitive automatic and involuntary movements help the developing baby to move through different stages of their physical development before birth, and play a particularly active part in the first two years or so of life.

- Reflexes are designed to provide a protective role for the baby over the first few months of life after birth as well as facilitating the different stages of early motor development: for example, grasping, rolling, sitting, crawling and gradually progressing to standing.

- These primitive or baby reflexes are normally inhibited by the maturing brain within the first year or two of life, although they can be elicited in older children and adults, and may re-emerge in an older person as brain inhibition becomes weaker.

- If these early reflexes are not inhibited and integrated by the brain at the appropriate stage, they may have an adverse impact not only on a child's motor development and the refining of movement, but also on motor skill acquisition.

The following reflexes, if still present in the school-age child, may also have an adverse impact on their higher functioning skills and educational ability. One or more reflexes noted below may be seen in the child with a developmental coordination disorder or motor dyspraxia and may have a particular influence on a child's school attainment (Goddard-Blythe, Beuret, & Blythe, 2017; see also the Institute for Neuro-Physiological Psychology in the 'Professional organisations' section):

- *Palmar reflex* – starts in the womb and is normally inhibited by four months.
- *Moro reflex* – starts in the womb and is normally inhibited by three months.
- *Asymmetrical tonic neck reflex (ATNR)* – starts in the womb and is normally inhibited by six months.
- *Symmetrical tonic neck reflex (STNR)* – starts at six to nine months (pre-crawling) and is normally inhibited by nine to eleven months.
- *Spinal Galant reflex (SGR)* – normally inhibited around birth.
- *Tonic labyrinthine reflex (TLR)* – starts in the womb and is normally inhibited by three to four months.

Palmar reflex

What: definition and meaning

What?

- The palmar reflex is a whole hand movement which emerges within the first 11 or 12 weeks after conception in the womb. Its function in part may be to help the baby maintain an automatic grasp – a 'safety' mechanism to enable the baby to hold onto the mother after birth.

- If the palm of a baby's hand is touched, stroked or has gentle pressure placed on it, the hand automatically closes into a fist with fingers bent. This response normally stays with the newborn baby during the first three months or so after birth.

- The palmar reflex should be automatically 'inhibited' within four to six months, allowing the baby to start to refine and isolate their finger and thumb movements in order to pick up and hold onto a small object with a 'pincer' grip using the opposing pads of the index finger and thumb.

- It takes a further few weeks for the baby to be able to release objects (hence the dropping of articles over the high chair) as this requires repetition and practice!

- Hand and mouth movements are strongly linked in the early years and are used for exploration of objects and the environment. In a newborn baby taking milk, a related 'kneading' movement of the hand may be noted as they suckle.

So what: issues and challenges

So what?

- Associated mouth or tongue movements may be observed when the child is writing, drawing or using scissors, particularly when the activity requires some resistance. This is due to the underlying retained hand and mouth neuro-developmental link. This associated movement is sometimes called 'overflow'.

- The child may have poor manual dexterity, as the whole hand grasp can limit independent finger and thumb movements. For example, in self-care activities, buttons, zips and scissor work will be harder for them and remain at a less mature stage of development.

◆ There may be lack of pincer grip, which can affect pen grip and control for cursive writing. The pen may be held in an immature position with the thumb lapped across the pen or with a general whole hand grasp making handwriting tiring and more effortful.

◆ Many children retain a palmar grasp if they are not assisted to refine their grip with fingers and thumb on the barrel of the pen, or move from a static pincer grip to a more dynamic active grip required for cursive writing. The immature pen grip does not, therefore, always reflect a developmental immaturity.

◆ The child may incur whole arm movements when writing, drawing or with general tool use, again making the activity far more effortful and extremely tiring when working for extended periods. They may be unwilling to write more than a sentence or two due to hand, arm, neck or back discomfort.

◆ The palms of the hand may be sensitive, making the child reluctant to engage in certain activities and withdraw from contact with certain materials and holding tools. Alternatively, some children with a palmar grasp often hold something in their hand at the expense of using that dominant hand to pick up an object.

◆ Speech and articulation may be poor and unclear due to the underlying link with hand and mouth that has not been automatically inhibited by the brain.

◆ Eating may be messy as the child does not have the musculature (oral motor control) for managing certain textures of food, and chewing takes longer.

◆ Certain foods may be harder to swallow; a stronger 'gag' reflex may be evident with a tendency for the child to choke. As a result, meals require more time and effort to deal with.

Now what?

Now what: practical strategies and ideas

● Provide a board angled at 20 degrees, angled desk or folder, for a correct upper trunk and forearm position. This allows the wrist to extend and the hand to fall into a naturally flexed position with the fingers and thumb coming together in a pincer grip action on the barrel of the pen.

- Encourage the child to place their index, second finger and thumb onto the neck of the pen, using a thicker barrel with an integral textured grip if necessary – a grip normally achievable by year one (see the 'Resources' section).

- Exercises can be provided under the remit of a practitioner specialised in the field of reflex integration, or a therapist with understanding of reflex inhibition/integration. See the hand exercises below – incorporate grasp and release exercises, progressing to isolating finger and thumb movements.

- Advice can also be sought from an occupational therapist on activity ideas to help desensitise the child's hands.

Activities to promote pincer grip and isolation of finger and thumb movement:

- Drawing on an upright chalkboard automatically assists the wrist and hand to fall into a pincer grip and correct wrist position (use chunky chalks).

- Encourage pincer finger and thumb grip using peg games; encourage wrist extension, and ensure that the child places the end pads of the index finger and thumb together when picking up a peg or a small object.

- Assist finger and thumb movements by incorporating pinch pots using clay and dough, activities using tweezers to pick up small objects, rolling marble/dice between finger and thumb, and turning pennies in the palm of the hand.

- Roll up a crepe bandage with one hand at a time using individual finger and thumb movements.

- Crumple up individual sheets of an old catalogue or telephone directory (use for target practice) – this provides strong 'grasp and release' exercise.

- Hit and keep a balloon in the air with a bat; once achieved, the child can then hit the balloon on alternate sides of the bat by turning the hand palm up and then back. Encourage the child to keep their elbow bent, to isolate forearm and hand movements.

- Playing the piano, flute or other musical instrument can help the child to refine and isolate individual finger and thumb movements.

- Keyboard training can be undertaken for children from the age of 9 or 10 if they experience ongoing difficulties with handwriting. A laptop can then be integrated into course work and examinations at secondary stage. Typewriting can be an additional remedial tool for finger and hand control, and in some children it can improve handwriting and spatial awareness in the recording of written and drawn information.

● Mouth control exercises – for example, blowing bubbles, suck and blow games – can be advised by a speech and language therapist, and additional advice can be sought from the same source if chewing, swallowing and speech articulation are adversely affected (see Royal College of Speech and Language Therapists in the 'Professional organisations' section).

Moro reflex ('flight, fight or fear' mechanism)

What: definition and meaning

What?

The Moro reflex is present as early as the first nine or ten weeks in the womb and is normally inhibited within two to four months in the young baby. It is elicited in response to an incoming, usually unexpected or unpleasant stimulus. It is there in part as a protective mechanism, and when stimulated can cause a whole-body movement and stress reaction in the body. In response, the baby may startle, fling their arms out to the side, bend both legs up into a flexed position, and take a large intake of breath prior to crying in a distressed manner.

The Moro reflex can be elicited by:

- A loud sound or noise – particularly if sudden and unexpected
- Bright light or other strong visual input or stimulation
- Sudden, unexpected movement or being poorly handled
- Pain or discomfort.

The consequences of a strongly retained Moro or 'flight, fight or fear' startle reflex may be observed in some children with autistic spectrum disorders who appear to be experiencing a high level of underlying stress. There may also be evidence of this reflex in some children with sensory processing difficulties who appear to be in a continual state of 'alert' with heightened sensory awareness.

The fear paralysis reflex closely links to the Moro reflex. Further reading is advised – see, for example, publications by child development expert Sally Goddard Blythe.

So what: issues and challenges

So what?

- ◆ In the older child or adult it is commonly termed the 'flight or fight' response, and puts the individual on high 'alert' with their focus on incoming peripheral stimuli at the expense of concentration and attention. It may be present in children with attention deficit hyperactivity disorder. This state may be a result of raised cortisol in response to a heightened stress and anxiety level. This is a normal mechanism but not if the child remains in this state; it is hard for them to relax with their 'sympathetic' nervous system in chronic 'flight or fight' mode.

◆ The child may have very tense muscles, particularly around their shoulders and back, commonly termed 'armouring'. They may be extremely sensitive to touch, especially if approached unexpectedly from behind. They may be intolerant of certain materials and be hypersensitive to a range of incoming stimuli.

◆ The child may be very sensitive to light – particularly fluorescent lighting – and find white interactive boards or paper too bright, which can then affect their response in class. They may rub their eyes, and find reading and writing tiring (see also the vision and eye movement control section in Chapter 4 for other causes).

◆ Visual perceptual problems may be evident, and the child becomes what is called 'stimulus bound': they are unable to screen out or ignore irrelevant visual material within their field of vision and focus on the peripheral information at the expense of the task in hand.

◆ There may be some auditory (listening) confusion as the child may be sensitive to a range of incoming sounds and be unable differentiate relevant input such as the teacher speaking over and above the sound of their peers.

◆ The child may find sleep difficult due to their hypersensitivity to sound and the general bodily discomfort experienced. The slightest sound may bring them up out of sleep, resulting in sleep deprivation for them – and those around them. It is not uncommon for these children to have night terrors and fear of the dark due to a very creative imagination.

◆ There is often a dislike of change, transition and surprises, and the child may be rigid and controlling in their daily lives to avoid changes in routine and therefore what is, to them, additional stress.

◆ Balance and general coordination may be compromised, particularly in ball games. The child may turn their head or blink or avert their eyes when a ball is thrown to them as a result of the heightened protective mechanism and response.

◆ Motion sickness when travelling in a car is not uncommon. There may be fear of physical activity as a result of an underlying immature balance system.

◆ The child may have reduced stamina, energy and exercise tolerance, but at the same time may have periods of overactivity.

◆ The child may be emotionally volatile and overreact to situations and have a free-floating anxiety which does not have any obvious source but which is heightened when they are put under pressure.

◆ Intolerance to wheat, dairy and other foods may be present (see BANT and Nutrition Science in the 'Professional organisations' section) and the child's immune system may be weak, also resulting in allergies, skin sensitivity, ear and throat infections.

◆ The child's blood sugar may fluctuate more than other children's, causing them to become particularly irritable prior to meals.

◆ The child may react adversely to criticism as they lack an innate sense of integration; self-image may be poor and they may find it hard to adapt to new situations. Decision-making can be difficult.

◆ The child may feel the need to control and manipulate situations in a desire to cope with their own anxieties and insecurities. Alternatively, they may demonstrate a high level of dependency on those around them due to the non-specific anxiety experienced.

Now what: practical strategies and ideas

Now what?

● A supportive structure and routine should be in place both at home and in school, with an understanding of the heightened stress levels the child may be experiencing.

● Plan a routine wherever possible; give the child verbal cues and a few minutes' warning for any transition or change of activity.

● Periods of quiet should be built into the school day and home routine (this assists most children). Whole class teaching is effective when group work is not underway, as it allows focus and attention due to extraneous sound being minimised.

● In class, also minimise visual distractions where possible. Keep the environment immediately round the child uncluttered and organised. Ensure the child is facing the focus of teaching and not distracted by facing their peers, unless for specific group activities.

- Lighting should be balanced and low level if the child's stress levels are to be lowered. Avoid fluorescent lighting and provide breaks from interactive whiteboards if the child's stress appears heightened.

- Coloured overlays or glasses with softer lenses may help to avoid the sharp contrast of black print on white paper or from interactive boards and computer screens. Give regular breaks when using technology.

- Provide positive feedback for effort made, avoid confrontation with a child who is stressed, and avoid shouting as this aggravates the situation.

- Build on the child's self-esteem as above, and ensure success in areas which may not be obvious initially. The child may be gifted in certain areas and find new confidence in a hobby or activity which fully absorbs them.

- A visual perceptual assessment may help to evaluate the child's interpretation of symbols and ascertain whether or not there are aspects of their focus that are out of balance.

- Provide some differentiation in PE and games for balance and coordination challenges. Be aware that the child may find excessive movement frightening, also heights and other challenging movement experiences such as walking along benches in PE, and using escalators and, to a lesser degree, lifts.

- Adapt ball games to build confidence, starting with throwing and catching balloons, larger foam balls and beanbags to avoid eliciting a 'startle' reaction.

- Be aware of the child's lack of stamina and exercise tolerance, or alternatively provide outlets for movement opportunities which can burn off excess energy.

- Allow the child to pursue activities which they find relaxing on their return home; provide them with a slow release high fibre snack prior to placing any further demands on them. Time out, in terms of relaxation, is important.

- Ensure that clothes are non-irritating and avoid scratchy labels to limit the amount of distracting extraneous demands on the child.

- Avoid 'learned helplessness' if the child has a high level of dependency; work towards success in small steps in activities, and allow extra time for the child to try activities hitherto avoided by them through fear of failure. They may be helped by taking responsibility in a task for someone less able. A child with this physiological makeup needs to feel valued and needs more reinforcement than others to prevent future inappropriate behaviours.

- Allow, where possible, a relaxing period before the child's bedtime; minimise any television programmes which can adversely affect the child's already charged-up nervous system.

- Give time for the child to share their anxieties and plan positively for the next day. Plan positive and enjoyable activities for the child to look forward to at some part of the week.

- Advice should be sought from an occupational therapist experienced in sensory integration for a full evaluation of the child's 'sensory' profile and advice on a 'sensory diet' if issues continue to arise. A course of occupational therapy to address some of the above areas may be advisable.

- Children with allergies and intolerances may require the advice of a nutritional therapist to build up their immune system and to provide an adapted diet if necessary. Ensure that their blood sugar is maintained, avoiding sugary snacks and providing foods which have slow release nutrition. Also provide adequate drinking water throughout the day.

- A referral to an osteopath who can treat and reduce the child's sympathetic nervous system response may be valuable. This can assist the child's body to relax physiologically, and ensure there are no other bio-mechanical problems.

Further classroom strategies to minimise stress

The following are designed to help a child 'modulate' their behaviour and cope if they become overloaded with too much incoming stimuli.

- Allow the child to stretch and take some deep breaths before settling down to work. Firm pressure, attained by sitting down, placing their weight onto straight arms with hands placed on the chair at either side of the body, can provide soothing feedback and help the child to modulate their behaviour.
- Provide the child with an uncluttered desk in a less busy part of the classroom, but where they face the board and the focus of teaching.
- At the start of a lesson, give the child sufficient opportunity to organise their equipment and writing materials to avoid any stress and tension. Any organisational difficulties can heighten stress and the fear of not being in control throughout the school day.
- Provide clear instructions on the order of activities to assist the child to plan and stay on task appropriately. Gain eye contact where possible to help the child to focus.
- Break down an activity into manageable steps for a child who has difficulty in processing and executing ideas on paper. Demonstrate an activity and provide visual and auditory cues where possible.
- If the child is 'fidgety' and 'on the move', purchase a cushion which provides acceptable movement while sitting. Ensure that the chair height allows the child's feet to be placed firmly on the ground – weight bearing through the feet can provide firm pressure feedback. This in tandem with the adapted cushion can help the child to self-regulate their behaviour.
- Where possible, alternate movement opportunities with periods of sitting and concentration – for example, by allowing the child to give out paper.
- A visual timetable assists the child to have control over their day. Writing on a vertical chalkboard prior to writing on paper facilitates good posture, shoulder stability and increased feedback through the joints (proprioception).

- The provision of an angled board (see Back in Action, Posturite in the 'Resources' section) provides support and stability for the forearms and therefore improved hand and pen control.

- Water and high fibre snacks allowed at regular intervals can assist concentration. Chewing and eating (where appropriate) provides increased proprioception, which can help to calm the child. Nail biting may be a symptom of stress, but also a need for proprioceptive (calming) input – the two can be linked.

- Allow a strategy of time out if the child becomes overloaded with demands, frustrated or stressed – this can result in outbursts of anger.

- Be aware that some children find touch uncomfortable and distressing; allow personal space when moving around with other children to avoid a negative or inappropriate response.

Sleep strategies and ideas for the younger child

- Allow the child the opportunity for physical activity at the end of the school day to release any pent up energy or frustration. If the child has difficulty in settling down afterwards, ensure that they have calming time prior to preparing for bed.

- Avoid overstimulating activities such as tickling and chasing around unless on the child's terms, as this can easily overload a child with an immature nervous system, particularly if they have difficulty modulating their behaviour.

- Establish a manageable and practical bedtime routine – for example, a warm bath (lavender essence can be relaxing), a warm milk drink, and the opportunity to unwind, talk about the school day and any concerns they may have. Try, however, to end the conversation on an 'up' note!

- Children with dyspraxia often have a heightened perception of what is going on around them and may be very sensitive to visual information that would be 'filtered out' by another child. Ensure, therefore, that any unpleasant or unsettling viewing material is avoided on television and/or computer prior to bedtime.

- Ensure when reading a story that the content and illustrations are suitable and the storyteller's voice relaxed and low. The child can be helped to calm down by wrapping them around with a blanket or cuddling them, where appropriate, as firm pressure (not restraint) can soothe the nervous system (this takes about 10 minutes).

- Soothing music can be played at bedtime. The 'Sound Health' series recordings have specially designed tapes to provide 'physiological' relaxation (see Learning Solutions in the 'Resources' section).

- Consider using blankets instead of a duvet, as these can provide soothing firm pressure feedback and some children prefer the weight of blankets and being tucked in. (This is a form of 'swaddling' for children – but not restraint) A sleeping bag is a good alternative for cosiness as long as the child can climb in and out easily. Where possible, place the bed against a wall to give a greater sense of security. Night clothing should ideally be made of cotton to provide extra comfort.

- A pillow placed in the bed along the child's back can provide firm, soothing pressure and reduce fidgeting. A hot water bottle with a soft cover can provide physical comfort.
- Check that the bedroom is not too light or too dark, too cold or too hot – keep the child's feet warm with bed socks if their temperature fluctuates.
- Additional blinds or lined curtains can be helpful during the summer if the child is sensitive to light, but with a small low-level nightlight to minimise fear of the dark if they have an overactive imagination.
- Glow-in-the-dark non-spill feeder cups can be purchased to put by the bed/cot for younger children.
- A simple prayer may help the child to feel safe and comforted.

Asymmetrical tonic neck reflex (ATNR)

What?

What: definition and meaning

An ATNR is an automatic whole body movement pattern which emerges in the womb and remains present up to approximately six months after a baby's birth. This reflex may play a part in the birthing process as it causes a whole body rotation movement pattern when the baby turns its head from one side to the other. It may, therefore, assist the body to rotate when the baby moves down the birth canal.

A 'fencing' or 'archery' posture can be observed in a small baby. It is elicited when the baby turns their head to one side – the arm and leg on that side stretch out and extend while the opposite arm and leg flex (bend). The opposite pattern occurs when the baby turns its head to face the other way. If this movement pattern is not automatically inhibited by the brain within the first year of life, the older child may have difficulty isolating head, body and arm movements in order to refine their arm and hand control. This particular reflex, if retained, appears to be linked with a lack of integration of both sides of the body (bilateral integration). Also it may limit the ability of the child to work across the midline of their body.

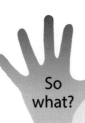

So what?

So what: issues and challenges

◆ The child may not have a clear hand dominance and may have a tendency to change hands during a task (mixed laterality). When undertaking more formal activities, the writing hand may not always be the most dextrous in some fine motor tasks (in other words, they are ambidextrous).

◆ Two-handed activities may be difficult for the child to coordinate – for example, in design and technology work, doing up laces and buttons, using a knife and fork – as they may not have a preferred leading or stabilising hand.

◆ The child may find it difficult to write and work across the body midline, and may twist or rotate their body or lean to one side to avoid it – this is usually done unconsciously, but more effort is incurred, making writing more onerous and less smooth.

- Excessive or fluctuating pressure on pen grips and paper may be noted: hand, arm and shoulder may ache due to the pressure exerted. (This may also be due to reduced body awareness and reduced feedback from the child's arms – see the section on proprioception in Chapter 3.)

- The child may have difficulty following a moving object in the horizontal plane with their eyes (visual tracking) and blink their eyes at their body midline due to poor integration of both sides of their body. Reading, including the ability to maintain line position and keep their place, may be affected. Words and letters may appear to 'jump around', or in some instances they may experience 'double vision'.

- There may be no clear eye dominance and the child may be unsure which eye to use when looking through a telescope or camera.

- The child may have a fluctuating profile with regard to visual perception, particularly when matching symmetrical shapes and figures.

- Balance may be affected when the head is turned from side to side, as whole body rotation may be elicited by the head movement and throw the child off balance.

- Difficulty with reciprocal cross-pattern movements may be experienced by the child during, for example, skipping, cycling and 'marching' patterns or when following a sequence of movements.

- When eating, the child may raise their elbows in the air at either side of the body as a result of the retained whole arm movement patterns. Use of knife and fork may be awkward with difficulty in cutting and controlling food.

Now what: practical strategies and ideas

Now what?

- Position the child facing the teacher and board or the focus of activity to limit the whole body rotation caused by turning their head. Handwriting and recording output will otherwise be adversely affected.

- Observe which hand the child tends to use as the leading hand for picking up and using a pen or object, and encourage the use of a consistent hand by placing activities to that side in the younger child.

- Encourage the child's wrist extension and dynamic tripod grip with the first two fingers and thumb placed on the barrel of the pen. A tripod grip allows use of the intrinsic, small muscles of the fingers and thumb for cursive writing. Exercises under the direction of an occupational therapist can assist the child to isolate head, trunk, arm, forearm, hand and finger movements to facilitate this skill.

- Provide the child with integral soft pen and pencil grips to ease pressure on the hand and fingers.

- Provide short breaks when writing for extended periods, 'shake' wrists and hands to relax and ease pressure, and provide an angled folder or angled posture board to rest the wrist on.

- Pen control is assisted by the child being placed symmetrically at the desk, with the height just below or at elbow level. Chairs which provide an upright position with lumbar support, allowing them to sit with their hips at 90 degrees for maximum stability, should be provided.

- Allow additional space on a shared table if the child tends to lean or shift to one side when writing to avoid crossing their body midline.

- Place the writing paper on the side of the child's writing hand; this can limit their need to write across the body midline.

- Provide the child with additional time to ease hand discomfort in tests and examinations.

- With the young child, practise tasks and activities which require both hands to be used together (symmetrical use); using both sides of the body together assists integration prior to working with cross-pattern movements. Use cooking, collages, crafts, construction and lacing games.

- Use paper with carbon backing to check the pressure exerted on the paper, which the child can see and then adjust. Extra paper under the writing sheet can also ease the pen grip and hand pressure.

- Formal keyboard training may be required prior to or at secondary stage if handwriting continues to be a real issue. The introduction of a laptop may be recommended by an educational psychologist or occupational therapist into appropriate lessons for the child to ensure competency prior to any of the key examinations.

- It is important to check functional vision with an optometrist (see BABO in the 'Professional organisations' section) if the child is experiencing strain and difficulty with maintaining visual focus on the board, at the desk or for reading.
- A comprehensive visual perceptual and visual motor assessment may be required by an educational psychologist or occupational therapist (see the 'Professional organisations' section). Activities can also be provided by a suitably qualified occupational therapist, following a comprehensive assessment, with advice and strategies provided which can be shared with the school.
- Therapy programmes for reflex inhibition can be provided by appropriately qualified therapists to assist in facilitating higher level functional skills (see INPP in the 'Professional organisations' section).

Symmetrical tonic neck reflex (STNR)

What?

What: definition and meaning

- A retained STNR may be present in children with a developmental coordination disorder or motor dyspraxia.

- It is one of a cluster of reflexes or involuntary automatic movement patterns, some of which emerge in the womb. The STNR normally presents after birth around the first six months of a baby's life.

- This reflex, which is part of normal physical movement development, helps the child to move into a four-point kneeling position prior to establishing crawling.

- If the reflex is retained after nine or ten months of life – around the usual period for crawling – it may have an adverse or 'blocking' effect on the progression of the child's motor development, affecting, for example, their ability to move forward and integrate left and right sides of the body for crawling.

- Crawling (using arms and legs in a reciprocal movement pattern) is an activity which may assist in maturing and integrating the following aspects of development and sensory motor integration:

    (a) The body's ability to perform reciprocal movement patterns and integration of both sides of the body (bilateral integration).

    (b) Eye and hand coordination and adjustment of eye movements near and far.

    (c) Postural stability – shoulder and hip strengthening while weight-bearing through shoulders and hips.

    (d) Feedback back through firm pressure for body position awareness (proprioception).

    (e) Wrist, finger and thumb extension (web space) for manipulation.

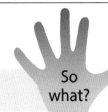

So what?

So what: issues and challenges

◆ The child may have never crawled using both sides of the body in a reciprocal movement pattern on all fours, preferring to bottom shuffle or 'commando' crawl.

◆ Where the STNR is retained, it can be activated when the child bends their head over their work at school, and their arms may automatically flex as a result of the linked movement which has not fully dissociated. At the same time the child's legs may have a tendency to straighten. The opposite pattern of movement can also occur, and the child may find whole body extension or flexion difficult, especially when sitting for long periods in a flexed position.

◆ As a result, it may be difficult for the child to maintain an upright sitting posture at a desk or table. They may 'prop' their head on their hand at the expense of stabilising their work or using both hands together, fidget, wrap feet behind chair legs, prefer to sit on their feet, and need change their position frequently. When in class the child may sit with their arms crossed and their legs stretched out in front of them (this posture can look oppositional). They may even try to stand up to write or lean back and write with their arms extended in an attempt to ease their postural discomfort.

◆ The child may find sitting cross-legged on the floor difficult and prefer to sit in a 'W' position with their knees bent under them, feet out to the side.

◆ They may dislike and avoid writing as it requires extra effort. Poor letter formation and excessive pressure on the paper may be observed, and they may break pencil points frequently. Discomfort in the neck, back and writing hand may be experienced.

◆ Homework can become a battlefield with the child. It may be rushed and the child may find it difficult to complete.

◆ The child may lose their place when copying work from a board or book in part due to difficulty with eye movement control and adjustment from one place to another (see advice on optometrist below).

◆ Reading difficulties may be experienced.

◆ Difficulty with maintaining attention may be experienced, with trouble focusing on a task. They may daydream, lose attention quickly, be easily distracted and fiddle with everything on their desk.

◆ Coordination challenges may be experienced by the child, especially between the upper and lower parts of the body, and they may have trouble with cycling, skipping, marching, running, catching and throwing; they may avoid certain sports as a result. Symmetrical activities such as skiing may not be a problem, and the child may be competent overall in these areas.

◆ When swimming using the breast stroke, the child may find it difficult to keep their head above water when bending their arms due to the linked head and arm flexion patterns.

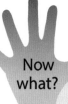

Now what?

Now what: practical strategies and ideas

● Allow some stretching and movement prior to sitting for extended periods, but also short appropriate movement breaks during the writing session to ease mechanical discomfort.

● The child may require a physiotherapy or osteopathic check to ensure that their spine is in alignment if they complain of back and neck discomfort when writing for extended periods.

● Encourage the use of an angled board or folder when writing to ensure that the upper body is as upright as possible – when the head is bent over the desk, the weight on the neck can change from approximately 4 kilos to 14 kilos due to the pull of gravity.

● Be aware that handwriting and schoolwork may be more laborious for these children than for their peers. Ensure that the child is facing the focus of teaching and notes are provided on the child's handwriting side where possible.

● Provide the child with integral pen grips to ease pressure as well as short breaks with additional time for written work as appropriate.

● Ensure a good visual line for copying from the board. Give the child time to adjust their vision from board to book.

● Check functional vision/eye movements with an optometrist to ensure eye strain and visual tracking are not a problem. This needs to be in addition to an optician's report (see BABO in the 'Professional organisations' section). Eye exercises moving eyes from near to far points and back may be helpful.

- Good postural support needs to be provided for homework, with opportunities for five-minute movement breaks from the work station. A higher stool and raised work surface or an angled cushion (Move 'n' Sit – see Back in Action in the 'Resources' section) may ease mechanical discomfort.

- Provide enhanced access to computers and/or a laptop for extended written assignments.

- Assess for the use of a personal laptop if the issues are causing real concern with regard to a mismatch between writing output and the child's innate skills. For example, keyboard programme information is available from IANSYST Ltd (see the 'Resources' section), and access should be sought for formal keyboard training to be integrated into school lessons prior to secondary school examinations.

- Upper and lower body coordination may be difficult, so some allowance should be given for games and PE activities which incorporate reciprocal movement patterns.

- Exercises to encourage total flexion/extension patterns may be helpful. A remedial exercise programme may be advised by an occupational therapist. For example, extending the full body in a slow stretch and then full flexion of the body, rolling it up into a ball and then stretching out, moving from the crouch position into a 'star' position. Exercises should be undertaken for 10 to 15 minutes, two or three times a week, and where possible be built into PE sessions.

- Specific swimming training may be required to assist the child to overcome the retained whole movement patterns of upper and lower body incurred by the retention of this reflex.

Activity ideas to assist large motor and reflex integration

All motor activities should be undertaken SLOWLY AND UNDER CAREFUL SUPERVISION.

- Wall push-ups. Stand at arm's length from the wall, heels down on the ground. With straight arms and wrists extended, place palms of hands flat against the wall while keeping back straight. Take weight onto hands, bend arms slowly and straighten – feel stretch on back of legs as arms are bent. Repeat five to ten times.

- Stand with arms out to sides; slowly turn body a full circle and then turn the other way. Repeat two or three times but monitor for dizziness and/or unsteadiness.

- Lie on stomach and lift head, chest, arms and legs off the ground as straight as possible for up to 30 seconds (if over the age of 7).

- Lie on back, reach out for and touch foot with hand on same side of the body. Change sides and repeat five times. Touch foot with opposite hand five times, change to other hand and foot and repeat five times.

- Lie on back, lift opposite legs and arms one at a time and then together, change sides and repeat. Lift alternate arms and legs in sequence. As one arm or leg is raised, lower the other one.

- Lie on back and reach for beanbag or half-kilo weight on opposite side of the body, pick up and place it on near side. Repeat with the other arm five times.

- Lie on back with arms and legs straight. Turn head to the left while slowly bending left arm and leg, then relax. Turn head to the right – slowly bend right arm and leg, then relax. Repeat both five times.

- Kneel on all fours, place left hand on left hip, turn the head to the left and lift and straighten right leg in the air, hold position to count of five. Repeat on opposite side. This may take considerable effort at first. *Work within the child's comfort zone in this and all the other advisory activities.*

- Lie in an extended position, roll slowly one way and then back again across floor mats.

- Kneel on all fours; with helper pushing against shoulders, crawl as far as possible and back again.
- Sitting cross-legged, plan a sequence of movements to include 'cross-pattern' clapping movement patterns incorporating working across the body midline. The child can make up or follow different sequences.
- Lie on top of a 'peanut' shaped therapy ball and gently rock onto extended arms and hands; allow arms to bend slowly, straighten and then roll back again. Stretch legs out straight when rolling over onto hands.
- Sit back to back against a large therapy ball with a partner – gently bounce back against the ball to gain firm pressure feedback while maintaining the sitting position.
- Sit with knees bent and pass a foam ball in figure of eight around and under legs, ensuring that the ball is passed across from one side to the other in order to work across the body midline. Take turns to plan different short sequences.
- Sit in a circle. Make a shape with hands and fingers, and 'pass it on' to the next person – each child to think up a pattern.
- Make a shape with the body and 'pass it on' to the next person – involve every child in the motor planning of the shape by giving each of them a chance to think up and demonstrate a new position.
- Dough, lacing and peg games can enhance pincer grip and isolate finger and thumb movement.

Spinal Galant reflex (SGR)

What?

What: definition and meaning

The spinal Galant reflex (SGR) is often associated with attention deficit hyperactivity disorder (ADHD), as it is known as the wriggling reflex. It usually integrates as the baby comes down the birth canal and is usually inhibited around birth. If not integrated as it should, the SGR can have an impact on the child's ability to sit still and focus in class or at meal times.

So what?

So what: issues and challenges

If the SGR is retained, the following issues may be noted in the child:

◆ Difficulty sitting without fidgeting, especially for extended periods.
◆ Dislikes light pressure on the lower back due to increased sensitivity, although firm but gentle pressure can over-ride this, so certain clothes will be preferred.
◆ Wetting the bed.
◆ Reduced concentration.
◆ Retaining short-term memory.
◆ There may be indication of hip rotation when walking.

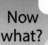

Now what?

Now what: practical strategies and ideas

● Us a sensory integration programme if possible.
● Snow angels: the child lies face-up on a mat or flat surface with his legs extended and arms at the side of his body. The child should breathe in and simultaneously spread legs outward and raise arms out along the floor and overhead, with the hands touching. The hands should touch at the same times the legs are fully extended. Exhale and return to the original position. The key is to get the child to move all four limbs slowly at the

same time. This exercise should be done five times several times a day until you notice that the child is fidgeting less.

- Twister game.
- Sit on a Move 'n' Sit air cushion or physio ball, starting with a few minutes at first and gradually increasing the time.
- Sit on the floor and walk forward and backwards on the buttocks.

Tonic labyrinthine reflex (TLR)

What?

What: definition and meaning

The tonic labyrinthine reflex (TLR) emerges in utero around three to four months and should integrate at three to four months after birth. This reflex links the vestibular (balance) sense to the proprioceptive (sense of body in space) and develops a sense of balance. If this is not integrated it will impact on integration of ATNR and STNR.

So what?

So what: issues and challenges

If the TLR is retained, the following issues may be noted in the child:

◆ Reduced static and/or dynamic balance, hunched posture.
◆ The child may have problems with judging space, distance, depth and speed. This may impact functional tasks such as riding a bike and looking up from paper to the board at school.

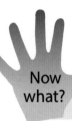

Now what?

Now what: practical strategies and ideas

Specific exercises aimed at the child feeling comfortable with looking down and up are recommended. The following beanbag games may be helpful (tip: start with sitting on the floor then progress to kneeling and then eventually standing):

● Put a beanbag on the head.
● Place hands, palm up, overlapping in front of tummy button.
● Without moving the trunk, tip the head forward and allow the beanbag to slide off.
● Catch the beanbag in cupped hands (most important action is the tipping action).
● Tip up to 10 times forward.
● Repeat the same actions BUT place the hands together at the back of the spinal area.

- Tip the head backwards – up to 5 times; ensure there is no discomfort.
- Try and increase the challenge with eyes closed, which may make the child a little unsteady. Some children compensate for poorer balance with their vision, therefore monitor.

Chapter 8

Daily living (self-care) skills

Independence in toileting

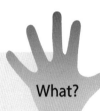

What: requirements for managing the toileting process

What?

- Awareness of body and limb position in space (proprioception).
- Reasonable range of arm movements.
- Manual dexterity and grip, the ability to manipulate fastenings.
- Tactile (touch) awareness when hands are outside the field of vision.
- Reasonable postural stability and balance.
- Basic upper arm strength for pulling trousers or underwear up and down; ability to hold dress or shirt up, and balance on toilet.
- Ability to reach toilet roll easily, manipulate paper, balance, and ensure clothes are out of way.

So what: issues and challenges

So what?

- The child may have a reduced sense of their own body scheme and limb position in space, adversely affecting their ability to carry out the activity effectively.
- The child may not be able to sense where their arms and hands are when outside their visual field (reduced proprioception).

◆ The presence of retained immature reflex movement patterns may affect manual dexterity and the child's ability to handle and manipulate toilet paper effectively.

◆ Balance may be poor when turning around or leaning over. The child may experience a feeling of being unsafe if their feet are not supported on the ground or on a small footstool due to postural instability.

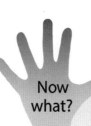
Now what?

Now what: practical strategies and ideas

● Inform the school's special needs or inclusion coordinator of possible problems to enable appropriate monitoring.

● Assist the child to follow the same routine where possible at home, which can also be translated into the school situation.

● Allow enough time for toilet routine – pressure will only aggravate the problem and create anxiety in the child.

● With a younger child, practise the routine at home, gradually reducing help as independence improves.

● Make sure the younger child's feet are supported when sitting at the toilet to provide postural security. If necessary provide a stable foot rest.

● Use a toilet seat insert for the younger child if postural stability or balance is poor.

● Toilet paper must be close enough with the use of a holder which allows sections of paper to be pulled off one or two handed.

● Disposable cleansing tissues can assist and be used in conjunction with toilet roll and kept by the child for use at school.

● Routinely reinforce the need for the child to wash and dry their hands properly.

● Where a child is reluctant, provide a star chart at home to note progress and effort made. Reward at the end of the week for a successful outcome as this can be motivating.

● Give praise and positive reinforcement for effort made, even if end results are not perfect (yet)!

Dressing skills

The following are approximate age guidelines for dressing skills.

At 1 year:

- Child can start to join in and co-operate when being dressed by holding out a foot or arm to push into shoe or armhole.
- Can pull loose socks off and start to pull at shoes to take them off.
- Can take or pull hat off.
- Some awareness of nappy soiling from approximately 15 months and may indicate this to the carer.

At 2 to 3 years:

- Can remove a simple item and shoes if article is undone or loose.
- Can place their foot into trousers, but not usually aware of correct leg.
- May help to push clothing down at the toilet.
- Can find armholes in a simple top with slight prompts and supervision.
- Will try to put on socks, also shoes and boots, providing balance is reasonable.
- Can put on a simple jumper or coat with help.

At 3 to 4 years:

- Starts to put on top – sometimes the wrong way around or inside out – may need help to position it and then take it off.
- Can pull lower looser garments down for toilet and, when changing, take them off.
- Should manage large buttons and can put shoes on with adapted fasteners, but not always on the right foot.
- Zips can be pulled up but needs help to insert the shank first.
- Starts to put clothes on the right way around with some exceptions.
- Fastenings become easier, including buttons and undoing front fastening zips.

- Gloves with fingers need help but can manage fingerless gloves and own boots.
- Can now dress but with prompting and supervision.

At 4 to 5 years:

- Should be able to achieve most fastenings with some help and guidance, including a zip.
- Can put socks on correctly and shoes with easy fastening should be manageable with a little supervision.
- Now technically old enough to manage laces!
- Should know the spatial orientation, back and front, of a garment.
- The child is on the way to independent dressing with prompts and some practical help.

At 5 to 6 years:

- Now should be able to put garments on the right way around and dress themselves unsupervised.
- Also, able to tie knots, including behind their back outside their visual field.

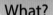

What?

What: requirements for competent dressing skills

- A reasonable sense of one's own body scheme and position of body parts (proprioception).
- A spatial awareness of personal body scheme in relation to the surrounding environment and clothes – what is up and down, side to side, in front and behind.
- Adequate sense of touch (tactile) feedback – not over- or under-sensitive.
- Reasonable hand and eye coordination, especially for fine motor tasks.
- Good balance and postural stability to be able to stand on one leg when putting pants or socks on and taking them off.
- Ability to work across the body midline when reaching across to position clothes and tuck them in.

So what: issues and challenges

So
what?

- ◆ The child may have a poor sense of their body scheme and be unsure which way to put their clothes on and how. They cannot organise their clothes when outside their visual field, leaving clothes untucked and generally untidy or out of place.

- ◆ Clothes may be put on back to front or inside out by the child; extra time may be needed to get clothes on properly. Sequencing, planning and general organisation for getting dressed in the morning, or for gym and sports, are difficult and frustrating for both child and supervisor. The child may seem 'all fingers and thumbs'.

- ◆ The child may be touch sensitive and, as a result, materials, labels, fastenings, waistbands may feel prickly and uncomfortable. The child will be constantly adjusting their clothes or fidgeting very often at the expense of focus on a main task.

- ◆ Alternatively, the child may lack touch sensitivity and be unaware of clothes hanging off their shoulders, poorly tucked in or not positioned correctly. They may not notice if shoes/boots rub and cause blisters.

- ◆ The child may become frustrated with fastenings and zips and become angry at themselves and those around them when struggling with getting dressed. They may avoid getting dressed and try to divert from the job in hand.

- ◆ Standing to get dressed may be difficult for the child if their static and moving balance is weak, their muscle tone 'low'.

- ◆ The child may not be able to coordinate both sides of the body properly for use, and have difficulty reaching across the middle of their body to put on and adjust clothing.

Now what: practical strategies and ideas

Now
what?

- ● It may assist the younger child with dyspraxia to engage in 'push–pull' games and activities or 'bounce' on a therapy ball prior to getting dressed, as this will give them increased sensory feedback and enhance their body position awareness (proprioception).

- At home, assist the child to prepare and lay out their clothes the night before. Establish a routine with drawers labelled correctly for socks, shirts and underclothes. Place clothes correctly in position, face down on the bed, to help the sequence and orientation of the garments in relation to the child's body.

- Use pictures or a wall-mounted poster of dressing and/or grooming sequences (teeth-cleaning, hair-combing), so the child can refer to that, in order to check and learn what to do next. You could make your own sequencing pictures, which might be fun to do together. As an example of 'ready-made' sequencing pictures, Orkid Ideas have some nice examples (see the 'Resources' section). They also have a system called Tom Tags that are helpful for packing school bags (and remembering what is needed to take and bring home).

- Provide a chair which offers more stability than a soft bed to limit balance difficulties; the clothes can then be placed on the bed in front of the child in a daily routine.

- Provide clothes with minimal resistance to being pulled on, such as trousers with elasticated waists. Put loops inside waistbands to pull up on if hand grip is weak; sew in elastic shanks for sleeve buttons which can remain done up but expand to allow the child to push their hands through. A circular clip such as a key-ring can be inserted into a zip to improve the child's grasp.

- Use large textured buttons for easier manipulation where possible. Use 'tube' or heelless socks – fold or roll down sock and insert toe. Talcum powder can help socks to slip on and off if feet get hot and sticky. Purchase shoes with adapted but normal looking fastenings.

- Provide natural materials where possible, remove scratchy labels, and avoid tight waistbands to limit any overt touch sensitivity. Avoid harsh detergents, use a natural clothes softener.

- Prompt the child to check in a mirror before leaving the room to ensure clothes are in position.

- Provide a hook on the door to hang large garments on, ready for the morning. Ensure outdoor clothes are placed on a hook in the correct position at the front door the night before to avoid further frustration, with a set place for shoes and boots.

- Allow the child additional time to get dressed and undressed at school for games and PE by letting them go first in the queue.

- Shoelaces can be a real challenge for children with dyspraxia/ DCD. Velcro shoes are helpful for all younger children. There are different ways of learning to tie laces, including the 'bunny ears' method. YouTube is a good visual, Internet-based resource and has many examples to aid learning shoelace tying. Replacing conventional laces with discrete elastic ones has become fashionable, especially for use in trainers. There are plenty of suppliers, such as Hickies (see the 'Resources' section).

- Advice and practical help for daily living and self-care skills can be sought from an occupational therapist if the child continues to struggle with dressing. The occupational therapist can also advise on core stability and balance exercises.

Chapter 9

Additional exercises, activities and therapy

Activities to strengthen trunk, shoulders and hips, and to increase body awareness

Please note that the activities recommended in this chapter are advisory only. The safety of the children is the responsibility of the supervising carer or instructor.

For a child who lacks confidence in the use of equipment, use the playground or gym when it is quieter with fewer children to compete with. Give positive encouragement and praise for any effort the child makes. Ensure success with the 'just right' level of activity, which may mean that they need to start with a simple movement activity, building up to an age-appropriate skill level over a few sessions.

- Child lies on stomach over large 'peanut' therapy ball and takes their weight on their extended hands through slightly bent elbows and wrists – then slowly straightens arms, lifts head, and extends body and legs. Child gently rolls forward onto fully bent elbows, lowers head and shoulders towards ground, then extends up again. Child repeats several times if comfortable with this.

- Note: do not attempt 'wheelbarrow' activities with weight of child's body supported through arms and legs, particularly if child's joints are hyper mobile or if muscle tone and general postural stability are weak. Child should always have support under their body.

- Provide 'peanut' ball for child to sit on with legs either side and gently bounce. Once feeling balanced, child can throw and catch beanbag or balloon while balancing on ball.

- Child sits back to back with partner, pushing against them – they lean forwards and backwards in a smooth and symmetrical manner, taking turns to take weight of other person's back.

- Try same activity but with large therapy ball placed between backs of partners. They should maintain upright position and a balance of force between them.

- Child kneels in upright position and maintains position while throwing and catching large foam ball or patting balloon backwards and forwards with partner. Depending on level of ability, they may progress to throwing and catching a beanbag.

- Child kneels opposite partner and pushes against their extended hands while holding body in upright position; they must try to maintain stability.

- Wall 'push ups' – child stands at arm's length from wall. With straight arms and extended wrists, they place palms on wall, keeping body and legs straight, and bend elbows and slowly lean towards wall, then extend arms slowly until pushed back into upright position. Child starts with four or five pushes and builds up number as shoulders and back become stronger. When done correctly, there should be a gentle pull on the calves.

- For younger children, make up obstacle course which encourages crawling (reciprocal movement patterns), changes of direction, stretching, balance and body awareness feedback.

- Provide playdough or theraputty for the child to knead and work. Ensure there is plenty of resisted two-handed activity to build up shoulder strength – this can be achieved by the child standing at a table and pushing down on dough. Bread or pizza dough making is also good, if messier, but you get a reward at the end.

Occupational therapy 'Activity Box' for primary school children

These activities provide intervention for the following areas and can be adapted according to each child's level of ability:

- Postural stability and strength
- Muscle strength for both gross and fine motor skills
- Static and moving balance
- Ball and targeting skills
- Bilateral integration – working both sides of the body together and in alternating patterns of movement
- Working across the body midline
- Body scheme and position awareness
- Motor planning and organisation of movement
- Eye and hand coordination
- Manual dexterity and fine motor skills
- Motor and visual spatial skills
- Sequencing and left and right orientation
- A multi-sensory approach using body movement, touch, vision, hearing and speech
- Fun and the 'just right' challenge: positive praise should be given for effort as opposed to the end result.

Materials required:

- Children's safety scissors
- Paper, glue
- Adhesive tape for marking out lines on a level floor
- Beanbag (can be made up with dried beans sewn into different shapes such as a triangle, square and circle – can be numbered or lettered)
- Baton
- Hoop
- Balloons – ideally large size but blown up to three-quarter size for strength

- A foam ball and tennis ball
- Range of coloured paper straws – large width for cutting and threading
- Self-adhesive stickers
- Coloured pencils and thick marker for lines for scissor work
- Tracing paper
- Carbon paper
- Graph paper
- Lace with a hard tip
- Dough – made to recipe (playdough or theraputty)
- Dice.

The activities will require:

- Allocated space, up to three times a week
- Floor that allows lines to be taped on it
- Wall to bounce a ball against
- 'Record' book to note strengths and difficulties and any changes.

The materials should be provided in a kit and set aside from general toys and activities. The equipment should be used constructively for a 10–15–minute session at least three times a week. Ideally each session should incorporate all the following:

- A fine motor manual task
- Balance, hopping or jumping practised two or three times
- Activities to work opposite sides of the body together.

Activities for balance, postural stability and bilateral integration

The child can be assisted to balance by holding hands with a helper, progressing to independent balance over the run of exercises.

Tape a 4-metre line on the ground. The child to:

- Walk, placing feet alternately in front of each other along the line, slowly and carefully. It may assist the child if they are told to fix their vision on a point on the opposite wall.

- Slowly walk along the line, heel and toes placed touching each other along the line. Hold the child's hand if necessary for support and to facilitate success.
- Move down the line, placing one foot at a time on opposite sides of the line.
- Place two feet together, jump both feet apart on either side of the line and then back together again, alternating the action to the end of the line.

Tape a 1-metre by 1-metre right-angled cross on the ground

- With feet together jump in a clockwise direction in and out of the four different sections until back to the start. Repeat two or three times at a steady pace.
- Jump from side to side in the different planes – left to right, right to left, up and down, down and up. The helper reinforces the exercise verbally to support spatial awareness.
- Jump backwards over the lines landing with feet together round all four sections.
- Hop using preferred leg – in a *clockwise* direction into all four sections.
- Hop using opposite leg – in an *anticlockwise* direction into all four sections.

Activities for ball and targeting skills, and eye and hand coordination

These activities use a beanbag, foam ball and tennis ball. Always allow the child a few initial practices. The child to:

- Kneel facing a partner, sitting back on the feet, then throw or roll foam ball to each other using both hands – up to 10 to 15 times slowly and methodically, watching the ball as it rolls. The distance between the partners can be adjusted according to their skill level.
- Repeat activity, but one-handed for throwing or rolling, using the dominant (handwriting) hand. Encourage consistency with dominant hand use.

- Stand to throw and catch foam ball two-handed.
- Repeat actions using a beanbag until successful (they may need to start closer together, at a metre distance and gradually increase space).
- Practise bouncing a tennis ball with the dominant hand until it can be caught successfully with both hands at least six times in a row.
- Stand between 1 and 2 metres from a wall, throw the ball and allow it to bounce and be caught using two hands together, up to 10 or 15 times.

Baton activities for postural stability and trunk strengthening, bilateral integration and peer interaction

- Sit cross-legged opposite a partner and with two hands placed on a baton, pull backwards and forwards in a rhythmic manner, as though rowing a boat, taking the partner's weight as they lean back. Ensure that some resistance is felt through the arms and shoulders.
- Kneel opposite partner, sit on heels and gently push and pull on the baton while maintaining an upright position.
- Kneel up on one knee, push and pull gently against the baton, change legs and repeat.

Hoop activities for bilateral integration using reciprocal movement patterns, working across the body midline, sequencing, counting and peer interaction

- Standing opposite partner, hold a hoop horizontally, placing both hands palms down on the hoop. Move hoop through hands to the left by placing the right hand across and over the other hand, releasing it and then grasping it again – 10 or 15 times slowly. Repeat activity, this time moving the hoop through the hands to the right.
- Standing opposite partner, turn hoop slowly in a vertical position by placing one hand above the other on the hoop while moving it through the hands. One partner will be moving the hoop up

and over, and the other will move it downwards. Then reverse the pattern of movement by feeding the hoop in the opposite direction. Ensure that fingers are extended when letting go of the hoop.

Balloon activities for eye and hand coordination, timing, force, sequencing and counting

- Keep the balloon up in the air for as long as possible with both hands, individually or with a partner.
- Keep the balloon up in the air for as long as possible using a baton or table tennis bat with the dominant hand, then with both hands together.
- The balloon can be filled with a handful of lentils to give sound feedback and make it a little heavier.

Dice games for fine motor skills, manipulation, isolating finger movements, assisting pen control and manual dexterity

- Manipulate a dice between finger and thumb, moving it up to the tip of each finger and back to the palm. Practise with each finger one at a time.
- Place a dice in the palm of the writing hand, call out any number up to six, then manipulate the dice using fingers and thumb to the correct number.
- Throw the dice, noting the number on the dice, then hold up the same number of fingers (up to five, including the thumb!) shown on the dice; try to keep the remaining fingers bent in the palm of the hand.

Straws/scissors for early scissor skills, fine motor manipulation and oral motor activities

Note: safety scissors should be used, under supervision.

- Cut several paper straws into pieces. Keep elbows at sides and thumb on top when manipulating scissors on a table at elbow height.

- Thread cut pieces of straw onto shoelaces or fine cord.
- Use straw pieces to make a picture with glue.
- Card-cutting following different width lines, shapes, angles and patterns that have been pre-drawn or printed. Start with thicker, straight lines and progress to curved and angled finer lines. Ensure the thumb is placed in the top hole of the scissors.
- Using a simple animal or pattern shape cut from tissue paper, blow the shape through a straw along the floor and over a taped line to denote the finish. Blowing games can help with extension of the body while sucking games help with body flexion.
- Bubble blowing can also be used for promoting oral motor muscle strength and control of breathing in tandem with other activities under the direction of a speech and language therapist.

Self-adhesive stickers, tracing, carbon and graph paper for fine motor and manipulation skills, and spatial orientation on paper

- Use stickers to make own picture designs. Provide the child with support to encourage imagination and success with manipulation.
- When tracing, choose favourite pictures and outlines to trace and then colour in. This activity can provide successful results for children who find free drawing difficult.
- Place carbon paper between two sheets of paper; write or draw on the top sheet to practise creating an even pressure on the bottom sheet.
- A stylus can be used on a tablet to create pictures with thin and thicker lines, depending on the stylus control. Carbon paper is best for monitoring pressure; however, a tablet and stylus can help develop finer control and precision.
- Graph paper is useful for writing the body of a letter or number, playing 'hangman', colouring in squares to make different patterns, copying a prepared design – progress from simple to more complex shapes. There are a wide range of imaginative colouring books for children and adults, which vary in design and complexity. Choose an appealing book, cut a sheet out of the book (assistance may be needed). Place the sheet on to a table or sloped writing board.

Simple playdough recipe for strengthening muscles of the hand and improving manual dexterity

This playdough takes 10 minutes to make. You will need:

- 8 tbsp plain flour
- 2 tbsp table salt
- 60 ml warm water
- food colouring (optional)
- 1 tbsp vegetable oil.

1 Mix the flour and salt in a large bowl, and in a separate bowl mix together the water, a few drops of food colouring and the oil.
2 Pour the coloured water and oil into the flour mix and work together with a spoon.
3 Dust a work surface with a little flour to prevent sticking and turn out the dough.
4 Knead for a few minutes to make a smooth pliable dough.

Encourage the child to participate in this activity for 5 or 10 minutes each session, so that the making of the dough becomes a 'pre-cooking' fun activity. It can be made the day before and stored in an air-tight container. Alternatively, ready-made pastry can be used and then made or cut into shapes to be baked.

- Squeeze and roll out dough using both hands, make up coil or slab pots from cut-out rectangular or square shapes.
- Create own designs in dough and make animal models, coil or slab pots.
- Roll out dough and mark patterns on it using everyday implements such as either end of a fork or spoon, then dry and paint.

Horse-riding ideas for the child with developmental coordination disorder (DCD) and allied conditions

There are many benefits to horse-riding and it is suitable for all ages. It is advised that a qualified riding instructor is sought and that the child's DCD and/or sensory issues are disclosed. Then the instructor can tailor the session to the child's needs to ensure a positive experience.

- Supervised horse-riding provides firm pressure feedback (proprioception) through the sensory systems, and when undertaken in a calm and steady way can assist a child to relax. Body scheme and limb position awareness is alerted, assisting sensory integration.
- If the child is sensitive to movement (over-responsive), all activity on the pony should be monitored and taken at a much slower pace initially in order for them to feel safe – make the experience dignifying, the 'just right' challenge and fun.
- Faster trotting in a large circle is stimulating for the child; this and also turning in different directions will stimulate their balance systems and help a sense of integration with the firm pressure feedback from the pony, providing the child feels safe and supported.
- If the child is movement-seeking with an under-responsive system, they will be able to tolerate much more movement and activity in horse-riding, but again they need to be closely monitored.
- Changing direction at a walking pace, and more particularly when trotting, helps to stimulate the child's balance systems and in turn to mature a rider's postural reactions and ability to adjust their body in space.

Horse-riding can assist the following areas to develop:

- Postural reactions and adjustments and body stability.
- Head control.
- Muscle strengthening of the trunk and upper body, arms and legs.
- Release of tight muscles, particularly in the lower limbs, with the assistance of gravity.

- A sense of one's body position in space and general increased sense of 'self'.
- Relaxation through firm pressure feedback.
- General coordination of muscles including eye and hand coordination.
- Strengthening and helping to sustain grip.
- Functional eye movement control.
- Integration of both sides of the body and helping the child to work across the midline of their body.
- Sequencing, letter and number work when used in the riding lesson.
- Visual and motor spatial awareness, a general sense of orientation in space – may help to overcome dyslexic tendencies regarding balance input, sequencing and spatial orientation, for example.
- General planning and organisation of movement.
- Communication and vocalisation.
- Feeling in control of a situation when supported appropriately.
- Providing a fun activity whilst interacting with the pony/horse's movement.

Horse-riding can provide sensory integration input for the following areas:

- Touch
- Smell
- Hearing
- Body position awareness
- Balance systems
- Vision.

Horse-riding can also provide positive input for:

- Cognitive skills
- Emotional connection
- Self-confidence
- Concentration and focus
- Self-discipline
- Care and compassion for animals
- FUN.

Practical tips prior to a lesson

- Ideally, ask the riders and their helper/assistant to stand a little way from the mounting block and then instruct each rider to come up one at a time with their helper/assitant. This enables the rider getting on the pony to know who is giving the instructions and providing support and avoids confusion caused by background noise.

- One person at a time should give verbal guidance to avoid auditory confusion in the rider. The child otherwise may not know who is giving the instructions or whom to listen to.

- Use a low and well-modulated but clear voice to soothe any initial anxieties in the child, particularly in the initial stages.

- Being assisted and moved up into the saddle may be alarming for some riders with immature balance systems, and may result in some stress responses such as hand-flapping and loud vocalising.

- Give the rider time to settle and relax down into the saddle. If safe, allow the child's legs to rest down either side of the pony for a few seconds before assisting the feet into the stirrups.

- Assist the rider to place their hands down onto the pony and feel a sense of their connection with it, before asking them to follow instructions.

- Describe the pony – for example, its name and colour – so the rider is able to focus on the animal as opposed to any fears they may be experiencing.

- Lead the pony away from the mounting block and prepare the rider with some simple exercises while the rest of the group are still mounting their ponies.

Exercises on the pony prior to the group activity

A selection of the activities below can be made depending on the rider and the time available.

- Remember that ideally only one person at a time should be giving instructions to avoid confusion for the rider.

- After ensuring that the horse or pony is clear of any other animal, the rider can then undertake some simple exercises.

■ Gently take the hands of the rider and explain what is going to happen, then assist them to give their arms a gentle shake to ease any tightness and tension in the shoulders. The rider should then relax their arms back onto the pony's neck or saddle.

■ Encourage the rider with clear spoken prompts to give their arms a good stretch – ideally up above the head – gently two or three times. Then ask and assist the rider to stretch their arms out to the sides and back again, two or three times.

■ The rider rests their hands onto the reins and then leans forward and reaches towards the horse's ears with both hands (providing the horse tolerates this well), then rests back into the saddle.

■ Encourage the rider to cross their arms across their body and give themselves a 'big hug' – then stretch their arms out in front of them and repeat the big hug, reaching across their body midline.

■ Assist or ask the rider to cross their arms out in front of them and place either hand on the opposite side of the pony's neck – cross and uncross the arms two or three times (integration of both sides of the body).

■ The rider places their hands on the front of the saddle – encourage them to look up to the roof, gently stretching and extending their necks, then to turn their heads to look at one side helper and then the other side helper. (This helps to isolate head and body movements and to provide neck, back and shoulder release. In addition, it provides social interaction and preparation for the ride.)

■ Rider pats the pony and then prepares to join the shared lesson.For more information see the Riding for the Disabled Association's website (RDA in the 'Professional organisations' section).

Climbing ideas for the child with developmental coordination disorder (DCD) and allied conditions

Climbing is an accessible activity for people of all abilities, including children with DCD/dyspraxia. There are many physical benefits such as facilitating:

- Head control.
- Postural reactions and adjustments and body stability.
- Muscle strengthening of the trunk and upper body, arms and legs.
- Improved joint stability
- A sense of one's body position in space and general increased sense of 'self'.
- General coordination of muscles including eye and hand coordination.
- Strengthening and helping to sustain grip.
- Functional eye movement control.
- Integration of both sides of the body and helping the child to work across the midline of their body.
- Visual and motor spatial awareness, a general sense of orientation in space.
- General planning and organisation of movement.
- Feeling in control of a situation when supported appropriately.

Climbing also has positive mental health benefits such as providing a sense of self and relieving feelings of stress and worries. During a climbing task, focusing on the physical movements is required, taking the mind away from other thoughts about the day.

As with horse-riding, it is essential to have a qualified instructor who is fully aware of the child's physical and sensory needs. One-to-one sessions are best to ensure correct techniques and to build confidence.

Children with low tone and/or hypermobility in some of their joints will tire quickly. They need to have shorter sessions to begin with, until they build up both their skills and muscle strength. This will improve joint stability and core strength, as well as confidence.

Local leisure centres sometimes provide indoor climbing wall facilities. A good introduction is 'bouldering'. Bouldering requires the climber to establish confidence and technical competence by learning to climb sideways, taking height out of the situation. Moving sideways is easier than pulling up, and therefore ideal for beginners. There are centres across the country which have brightly coloured, engaging walls and vary in difficulty. Some of these centres provide dedicated time slots for children with specific learning differences. Reasonable adjustments are made, such as turning off the music, having fewer people in each session and increasing the staff to child ratio. This enables children with sensory sensitivities to participate comfortably, succeed and gain a sense of pleasure and achievement.

Resources

Note: all websites included here are correct at May 2019, but may be subject to change.

Afasic a Voice for Life – www.afasic.org.uk – website full of information and resources relating to language difficulties.

Ann Arbor Publishers Ltd – www.annarbor.co.uk – assessment materials and resources for special educational needs.

Anything Left Handed – www.anythingleft-handed.co.uk – help for left-handed children information page.

Back in Action – www.backinaction.co.uk – posture pack – a portable writing slope, seat wedge with pencil/paper storage and carry handle, Move 'n' Sit cushions.

British Dyslexia Association – www.bdadyslexia.org.uk – help with handwriting information page.

Cleverstix – www.cleverstix.com – child development cutlery.

Come Unity – www.comeunity.com – articles to help your child with sensory integration issues.

Crossbow Education – www.crossboweducation.com – resources for visual stress and other SEN resources.

Dyspraxia Foundation – dyspraxiafoundation.org.uk – UK national charity supporting those with dyspraxia. Wealth of information sheets for all ages.

Happy Puzzle Company Ltd – www.happypuzzle.co.uk – fun and educational activities and resources for schools.

Hickies – uk.hickies.eu – tie-free shoe laces.

IANSYST Ltd – www.dyslexic.com – whole range of IT and allied resources for children with dyslexia.

Incentive Plus Ltd – www.incentiveplus.co.uk – social, emotional and behavioural resources for children and young people.

LDA – www.ldalearning.com – full range of resources for primary school, including extensive handwriting materials, gross and fine motor equipment and materials.

Learning Solutions – www.learning-solutions.co.uk – therapeutic music to enhance development, health and functioning.

Orkid Ideas – www.orkidideas.com – TomTags visual support system to help children understand, follow and remember what they need to do.

National Handwriting Association – www.nha-handwriting.org.uk – a multidisciplinary group based in the United Kingdom. The association promotes the improvement of handwriting standards in schools and supports children with handwriting difficulties. Publications are available to EU and non-EU members. Also contains details of Handwriting Interest Group and membership application forms.

Pencil Grip – www.thepencilgrip.com – products include a range of pen/pencil grips and other resources.

PETA UK – www.peta-uk.com – provides a range of photocopiable resources for pre-scissor and scissor skills as well as a range of equipment.

Posturite – www.posturite.co.uk – includes writing slopes suitable for older children and adults.

ROMPA – www.rompa.com – products, services and concepts for people of all ages with sensory impairments and learning disabilities.

Sensory Integration – www.sensoryintegration.org.uk – committed to the promotion and development of sensory integration theory and practice.

Southpaw Enterprises – www.southpaw.com – offers sensory integration and developmental products, paediatric therapy equipment, resources and support for therapeutic professionals and health care professionals, schools and families.

SpaceKraft – www.spacekraft.co.uk – develops and manufactures a full range of sensory products for carers and teachers working with special needs children.

Special Direct – www.tts-group.co.uk/primary/sen-special-direct/ – handwriting, fine motor, self-esteem, emotional and allied resources.

Speechmark – https://www.routledge.com/posts/12301 – includes speech and language, emotional development, games and activities.

Taskmaster – www.taskmasteronline.co.uk – for a range of specialist equipment including adapted scissors kit.

TFH Special Needs Toys – www.specialneedstoys.com – a range of products covering physical play, relaxation and daily living activities.

Winslow Resources – www.winslowresources.com – resources and information covering a wide range of conditions.

Professional organisations

British Association of Behavioural Optometrists (BABO) – www.babo.co.uk – explains what behavioural optometry is and the role of vision in learning. Includes how to find a behavioural optometrist.

British Association for Nutrition and Lifestyle Medicine (BANT), 27 Old Gloucester St, London WC1N 3XX – www.bant.org. uk – professional body for nutritional therapists. Members are qualified in the science of nutrition and provide nutritional therapy.

British Chiropractic Association, 59 Castle Street, Reading, Berkshire RG1 7SN – www.chiropractic-uk.co.uk – for advice and assistance with back pain in children (which may be exacerbated by poor sitting positions in class, leaning over flat tables, twisting round in seats to see the teacher, as well as sedentary lifestyle and a lack of opportunity to build up core stability and muscles).

British Dyslexia Association, Unit 8, Bracknell Beeches, Old Bracknell Lane, Bracknell, Berkshire RG12 7BW – www. bdadyslexia.org.uk.

British Osteopathic Association (BOA), 3 Park Terrace, Manor Road, Luton, Bedfordshire LU1 3HN – www.osteopathy.org.uk – a UK professional association of osteopaths.

British Psychological Society, St Andrews House, 48 Princess Road East, Leicester LE1 7DR – www.bps.org.uk – includes a directory of chartered psychologists and covers all different specialisms, for example, education.

Chartered Society of Physiotherapy (CSP), 14 Bedford Row, London WC1R 4ED – www.csp.org.uk – the professional, educational and trade union body for chartered physiotherapists.

Dyspraxia Foundation, 8 West Alley, Hitchin, Herts SG5 1EG – www.dyspraxiafoundation.org.uk.

Dyspraxia UK – www.dyspraxiauk.com – occupational therapy service offering diagnostic assessments for all ages.

Independent Panel for Special Educational Advice (IPSEA), 6 Carlow Mews, Woodbridge, Suffolk IP12 1EA – www.ipsea.org.uk – including statementing of children with special educational needs.

Institute for Neuro-Physiological Psychology (INPP), 1 Stanley Street, Chester CH1 2LR – www.inpp.org.uk – a range of excellent publications on the impact of reflexes on childhood and education, practitioners and training for a range of developmental issues.

Mind, 15-19 Broadway, Stratford, London E15 4BQ – www.mind.org.uk – provide advice and support to empower anyone experiencing a mental health problem.

Movement Matters – www.movementmattersuk.org – UK umbrella organisation representing the major national groups concerned with children and adults with developmental coordination disorder (or DCD).

National Autistic Society, 393 City Road, London EC1V 1NG – www.autism.org.uk.

Riding for the Disabled Association (RDA), Lowlands Equestrian Centre, Old Warwick Road, Shrewley, CV35 7AX – www.rda.org.uk – an organisation with a body of volunteers who are dedicated to providing a range of services including riding tuition for children and young people with disabilities.

Royal College of Occupational Therapists (RCOT), 106–114 Borough High Street, Southwark, London SE1 1LB – rcot.co.uk.

Royal College of Occupational Therapists Specialist Section – Independent Practice (RCOTSS-IP) – rcotss-ip.org.uk.

Royal College of Speech and Language Therapists (England), 2 White Hart Yard, London SE1 1NX – www.rcslt.org – to find a speech and language therapist.

Recommended reading and references

Addy L, 2016, *How to Support Children with Sensory Processing Needs*, LDA Publications, Hyde, Cheshire.

American Psychiatric Association, 2013, *Diagnostic and Statistical Manual of Mental Disorders (5th ed.)*, American Psychiatric Association, Washington, DC.

Barsch R, 1995, *Fine Tuning: An Auditory-Visual Training Program*, Academic Therapy Publications, Novato, California.

Biel L & Peske N (Foreword by Grandin T), 2009, *Raising a Sensory Smart Child: The Definitive Handbook for Helping Your Child with Sensory Integration Issues*, Penguin Group, New York.

Biggs V, 2014, *Caged in Chaos: A Dyspraxic Guide to Breaking Free*, Jessica Kingsley Publishers, London.

Binnion J & Shelbourne C, 2017, *You're So Clumsy Charlie (Age 6 – 8 Years)*, Your Stories Matter, Lancaster.

Buzan T, 2005, *Mind Maps for Kids (9 – 12 Years)*, Thorsons Publication, London.

Christmas J, 2012, *Sensory Dinosaurs: A Speechmark Practical Therapy Resource*, Routledge, Abingdon.

Collins-Donnelley K, 2014, *Banish Your Self Esteem Thief: A Cognitive Behavioural Therapy Workbook for Young People*, Jessica Kingsley Publishers, London.

Collins-Donnelley K, 2019, *Starving the Anxiety Gremlin: A Cognitive Behavioural Therapy Workbook for Young People*, Jessica Kingsley Publishers, London.

Evans J & March R, 2017, *Vera McLuckie and the Daydream Club (Ages 7 – 9 Years)*, Your Stories Matter, Lancaster.

Gianetti M & Russita T, 2017, *Emily's Sister: A Family Journey with Dyspraxia & Sensory Processing Disorder (Ages 7 – 9 Years)*, Your Stories Matter, Lancaster.

Goddard-Blythe S, Beuret LJ & Blythe P, 2017, *Attention, Balance & Coordination: The ABC of Learning Success (2nd ed.)*, Wiley-Blackwell, Hoboken, New Jersey.

Hannell G, 2006, *Identifying Children with Special Needs: Checklists for Professionals*, SEN Marketing, Wakefield.

Hastings N & Chantrey Wood K, 2002, *Re-organizing Primary Classroom Learning*, Open University Press, Buckingham.

Kirby A & Peters L, 2020, *100 Ideas for Supporting Secondary School Children with Dyspraxia*, Bloomsbury Education, London.

Kranowitz C, 2005, *The Out-of-sync Child: Recognizing and Coping with Sensory Processing Disorder*, Perigee Book, New York.

Patrick A, 2015, *The Dyspraxic Learner: Strategies for Success*, Jessica Kingsley Publishers, London.

Sheridan M, 2014, *From Birth to Five Years: Children's Developmental Progress (4th ed.)*, Routledge, Abingdon.

Voss A, 2011, *Understanding Your Child's Sensory Signals: A Practical Daily Use Handbook for Parents and Teachers*, Create Space Independent Publishing Platform, Scotts Valley, California.

Walker S, 2015, *Waiting for a Voice: The Parent's Guide to Coping with Verbal Dyspraxia*, Emerald Publishing, UK Edition, Bingley.

Wing L, 2003, *The Autistic Spectrum: A Guide for Parents and Professionals (2nd ed.)*, Robinson Publishing, London.

World Health Organisation, 2018, *International Classification of Diseases (ICD) (11th Ed.)*, World Health Organisation, Geneva.

Index

Hands on
DYSPRAXIA

This updated new edition is a practical guidebook for parents, teachers and other professionals supporting children with sensory and motor learning difficulties. It offers an understanding of developmental coordination disorder (DCD), and the impact that this can have in both home and school settings. Each chapter offers practical 'hands-on' strategies, activities and ideas for managing the effects of the condition as well as providing a sound medical and physiological understanding of the condition to facilitate access to education and everyday living.

Each chapter contains:

- A clear explanation of potential challenges that people with DCD and coexisting conditions face, with an introductory definition, along with reference to current terminology
- Exploration of the implications of these challenges on home life, educational and social environments
- Practical strategies and ideas to help the child or young person reach their full potential

Written by occupational therapists with extensive experience of DCD/dyspraxia and possible associated conditions, this book is structured in an accessible way, suitable for: parents, carers, teachers or health professionals seeking guidance for the young people they support. This is a must read for anybody looking to support children and young people with this often misunderstood condition.

Though now retired as an occupational therapist, **Jill Christmas** still continues to provide informal advice to parents, grandparents and carers who have children struggling with issues caused by dyspraxia and allied challenges. Jill was previously the principal of her own clinic, which had a team of occupational therapists and other linked professionals. The clinic had contracts with Special Schools, LEAs and the NHS for the assessment and treatment of children with dyspraxia, DCD, A[DH]D, austistic spectrum disorders, sensory integrative dysfunction and a range of other conditions. The clinic now continues under different management and is based in Sussex.

Rosaline Van de Weyer has both a personal and professional interest in supporting people with DCD. Her son was diagnosed with DCD at the age of 8 years old. She experiences the joys and, at times, heartache of bringing up a 'distracted', 'needs to write more neatly' (school reports) fabulous young man. Occupational therapy has been a passion for 20 years, helping people overcome difficulties and thrive in all aspects of life. Rosaline manages Dyspraxia UK, an occupational therapy assessment service for people of all ages. This service is primarily independent, but is commissioned by NHS Clinical Commissioning Groups in areas that do not have existing services to meet the demand.